MW01275566

CORE CURRICULUM FOR
PROFESSIONAL EDUCATION IN PAIN

Mission Statement of IASP Press

The International Association for the Study of Pain (IASP) is a nonprofit, interdisciplinary organization devoted to understanding the mechanisms of pain and improving the care of patients with pain through research, education, and communication. The organization includes scientists and health care professionals dedicated to these goals. The IASP sponsors scientific meetings and publishes newsletters, technical bulletins, the journal *Pain,* and books.

The goal of IASP Press is to provide the IASP membership with timely, high-quality, attractive, low-cost publications relevant to the problem of pain. These publications are also intended to appeal to a wider audience of scientists and clinicians interested in the problem of pain.

Recent publications from IASP Press

Back Pain in The Workplace, Management of Disability in Nonspecific Conditions, Task Force on Pain in the Workplace, edited by W.E. Fordyce

Visceral Pain, edited by Gerald F. Gebhart

Temporomandibular Disorders and Related Pain Conditions, edited by Barry J. Sessle, Patricia S. Bryant, and Raymond A. Dionne

Touch, Temperature, and Pain in Health and Disease: Mechanisms and Assessments, edited by Jörgen Boivie, Per Hansson, and Ulf Lindblom

Classification of Chronic Pain: Descriptions of Chronic Pain Syndromes and Definitions of Pain Terms, Second Edition, Task Force on Taxonomy, edited by H. Merskey and N. Bogduk

Proceedings of the 7th World Congress on Pain, edited by Gerald F. Gebhart, Donna L. Hammond, and Troels S. Jensen

Pharmacological Approaches to the Treatment of Chronic Pain: New Concepts and Critical Issues, edited by Howard L. Fields and John C. Liebeskind

CORE CURRICULUM FOR PROFESSIONAL EDUCATION IN PAIN

a report of the

Task Force on Professional Education
of the
International Association for the Study of Pain

Editor

Howard L. Fields, MD, PhD
Departments of Neurology and Physiology
University of California School of Medicine
San Francisco, California, USA

IASP PRESS • SEATTLE

© 1995 IASP Press,
International Association for the Study of Pain

All rights reserved. No part of this publication may be reproduced, stored in a retrieval system, or transmitted, in any form or by any means, electronic, mechanical, photocopying, recording, or otherwise, without the prior written permission of the publisher.

No responsibility is assumed by IASP for any injury and/or damage to persons or property as a matter of product liability, negligence, or from any use of any methods, products, instruction, or ideas contained in the material herein. Because of the rapid advances in the medical sciences, the publisher recommends that there should be independent verification of diagnoses and drug dosages.

Library of Congress Cataloging-in-Publication Data

International Association for the Study of Pain. Task Force on Professional
    Education.
        Core curriculum for professional education in pain : a report of the Task
    Force on Professional Education of the International Association for the Study
    of Pain / editor, Howard L. Fields. -- 2nd ed.
            p.   cm.
        Includes bibliographical references
        ISBN 0-931092-12-4
        1. Pain—Outlines, syllabi, etc. 2. Pain—Study and teaching
    (Continuing education)   I. Fields, Howard L. II. Title.
        [DNLM: 1. Pain—outlines. 2. Education, Medical, Continuing—outlines.
    3. Curriculum—outlines.   WL 18.2 C797 1995]
    RB127. I56   1995
    616´ .0472—dc20
    DNLM/DLC
    for Library of Congress   95-44088
                                                              CIP

IASP Press
International Association for the Study of Pain
909 NE 43rd St., Suite 306
Seattle, WA 98105 USA
Fax: 206-547-1703

Printed in the United States of America

Contents

List of Members amd Consultants of the Task Force on
    Professional Education   vii
Foreword by Howard L. Fields   xi

1. Anatomy and Physiology   1
2. Pharmacology of Pain Transmission and Modulation   5
3. Pain Measurement in Humans   9
4. Psychosocial Aspects of Pain   13
5. General Principles of Pain Evaluation and Management   19
6. Designing, Reporting, and Interpreting Clinical Trials of
    Treatments for Pain   23
7. Drug Treatment I: Opioids   27
8. Drug Treatment II: Antipyretic Analgesics, i.e., Nonsteroidals,
    Acetaminophen, and Phenazone Derivatives   33
9. Drug Treatment III: Antidepressants, Anticonvulsants,
    and Miscellaneous Agents   37
10. Physical Medicine and Rehabilitation   45
11. Nonsurgical Peripherally Applied Neuroaugmentative and
    Counterirritation Techniques   49
12. Surgical Approaches   53
13. Nerve Blocks   59
14. Psychiatric Evaluation and Treatment   63
15. Psychological Treatments (Behavioral Interventions)   67
16. Multidisciplinary Pain Management   71
17. Taxonomy of Pain Syndromes   73
18. Low Back Pain   75
19. Myofascial Pain   79
20. Neuropathic Pain   83
21. Headache   87
22. Rheumatological Aspects of Pain   89
23. Cancer Pain   93
24. Postoperative Pain   99
25. Compensation, Disability Assessment, Pain in the Workplace   105
26. Orofacial Pain, Including Temporomandibular Disorders   109
27. Animal Models of Pain and Ethics of Animal Experimentation   111
28. Pain in Children   113
29. Ethical Standards in Pain Management and Research   117

Members of the Task Force
on Professional Education

Stephen E. Abram, MD, *Professor and Vice Chairman of Anesthesiology, Medical College of Wisconsin, Milwaukee, Wisconsin, USA*

Pedro F. Bejarano, MD, *Assistant Professor of Anesthesiology, Escuela Colombiana de Medicina, Pain Medicine Section, Department of Anesthesiology, Fundación, Santa Fe de Bogotá Santafé de Bogotá, Santafé de Bogotá D.C., Colombia*

Costantino Benedetti, MD, *Director, Anesthesia, Cancer Pain and Symptom Control; Director, Comprehensive Oncology Rehabilitation Program, The Arthur G. James Cancer Hospital and Research Institute; Professor, Clinical Anesthesiology, The Ohio State University Hospital, Columbus, Ohio, USA*

Gary J. Bennett, PhD, *Chief, Neuropathic Pain and Pain Measurement Section, Neurobiology and Anesthesiology Branch, National Institute of Dental Research, National Institutes of Health, Bethesda, Maryland, USA*

Aleksandar Berić, MD, DSc, *Director of Clinical Neurophysiology, Hospital for Joint Diseases; Associate Professor of Neurology, New York University Medical Center, New York, USA*

Jean-Marie Besson, DSc, PharmD, *Director, Laboratoire de Physiopharmacologie du Système, Nerveux, and Laboratoire de Physiopharmacologie de la Douleur, Paris, France*

David Borsook, MB, PhD, *Director, MGH Pain Center, Department of Anesthesia, Massachusetts General Hospital; Assistant Professor in Anesthesia (Neurology), Department of Anaesthesia, Harvard Medical School, Boston, Massachusetts, USA*

Kay Brune, MD, *Professor and Chairman, Department of Pharmacology and Toxicology, University of Erlangen, Erlangen, Germany*

Keith Budd, MB ChB, *Department of Anaesthetics, Royal Infirmary, Bradford, United Kingdom*

Rene Cailliet, MD, *Rehabilitation Medicine, Pacific Palisades, California, USA*

Daniel B. Carr, MD, *Saltonstall Professor of Pain Research, Professor of Anesthesia and Medicine, New England Medical Center, Tufts University, Boston, Massachusetts, USA*

Fernando Cervero, MD, DSc, *Professor of Physiology, Department of Physiology and Pharmacology, University of Alcala de Henares, Madrid, Spain*

Charles Chabal, MD, *Associate Professor of Anesthesiology and the Multidisciplinary Pain Clinic, University of Washington School of Medicine, Seattle, Washington, USA*

C. Richard Chapman, PhD, *Professor, Departments of Anesthesiology and Psychiatry and Behavioral Sciences, University of Washington; Director, Pain and Toxicity Research Program, Division of Clinical Research, Fred Hutchinson Cancer Research Center, Seattle, Washington, USA*

J. Edmond Charlton, MB BS, FRCA, *Consultant in Pain Management and Anaesthesia, Royal Victoria Infirmary, Newcastle upon Tyne, United Kingdom*

Kenneth D. Craig, PhD, *Professor, Department of Psychology, University of British Columbia, Vancouver, British Columbia, Canada*

Nance Cunningham, MA, *Adjunct Professor, Department of Philosophy, Oklahoma City University; Associate, Center for Health Policy Research and Development, University of Oklahoma Health Sciences Center, Oklahoma City, Oklahoma, USA*

Ronald Dubner, DDS, PhD, *Professor and Chair, Department of Oral and Craniofacial Biology, University of Maryland Dental School, Baltimore, Maryland, USA*

Samuel F. Dworkin, DDS, PhD, *Professor, Department of Oral Medicine, School of Dentistry, Department of Psychiatry and Behavioral Sciences, School of Medicine, University of Washington, Seattle, Washington, USA*

Howard L. Fields, MD, PhD, *Professor, Departments of Neurology and Physiology, University of California School of Medicine, San Francisco, California, USA*

Andrew A. Fischer, MD, PhD, *Associate Clinical Professor of Rehabilitation Medicine, Mount Sinai School of Medicine (CUNY); Chief, Physical Medicine and Rehabilitation Service, Veterans Affairs Medical Center, Bronx, New York, USA*

David A. Fishbain, MD, FAPA, *Professor of Psychiatry and Neurological Surgery, University of Miami School of Medicine; Liaison Psychiatrist, University of Miami Comprehensive Pain Center at South Shore Hospital, Miami, Florida, USA*

Herta Flor, PhD, *Professor of Clinical Psychology and Behavioral Neuroscience, Humboldt University, Berlin, Germany*

James R. Fricton, DDS, MS, *Associate Professor, Division of TMD and Orofacial Pain, Department of Diagnostic and Surgical Sciences, University of Minnesota School of Dentistry, Minneapolis, Minnesota, USA*

Phillip B. Gaukroger, MB BS, FANZCA, *Clinical Lecturer, University of Adelaide; Senior Consultant, Paediatric Anaesthesia and Pain Management, Women's and Children's Hospital, North Adelaide, South Australia, Australia*

Gerald F. Gebhart, PhD, *Professor, Department of Pharmacology, University of Iowa, Iowa City, Iowa, USA*

Hartmut Goebel, Dr Med, Dip Psych, *Noer, Germany*

Richard H. Gracely, PhD, *Research Psychologist, Neuropathic Pain and Measurement Section, Neurobiology and Anesthesiology Branch, National Institute of Dental Research, National Institutes of Health, Bethesda, Maryland, USA*

Ji-Sheng Han, MD, *Member of the Chinese Academy of Sciences; Director, Neuroscience Research Center; Professor, Department of Physiology, Beijing Medical University, Beijing, People's Republic of China*

Hermann O. Handwerker, Prof, Dr Med, *Professor of Physiology, Institute of Physiology and Experimental Pathophysiology, University of Erlangen-Nürnberg, Erlangen, Germany*

Malcom I. Jayson, MD, FRCP, *Professor, Rheumatology, Rheumatic Diseases Centre, University of Manchester, Hope Hospital, Salford, United Kingdom*

Kai Jensen, MD, DMSc, *Chief Neurologist, Department of Neurology, Hilleroed Hospital, Hilleroed, Denmark*

Ronald M. Kanner, MD, *Department of Neurology, Long Island Jewish Medical Center, New Hyde Park, New York; Professor of Neurology, Albert Einstein College of Medicine, Bronx, New York, USA*

Martin Koltzenburg, MD, *Department of Neurology, University of Würzburg, Würzburg, Germany*

Jon D. Levine, MD, PhD, *Professor of Medicine, University of California, San Francisco, California, USA*

John D. Loeser, MD, *Professor, Departments of Neurological Surgery and Anesthesiology, University of Washington School of Medicine; Director, Multidisciplinary Pain Center, University of Washington Medical Center, Seattle, Washington, USA*

Peter N. Malleson, MB, BS, MRCP(UK), FRCPC, *Associate Professor, Division of Rheumatology, Department of Pediatrics, University of British Columbia; Director, Children's Program, Arthritis Society (B.C. and Yukon), Vancouver, British Columbia, Canada*

Serge Marchand, PhD, *Director, Sciences Sociales et Sante, Université Québec, Rouyn Noranda, Quebec, Canada*

Mitchell B. Max, MD, *Chief, Clinical Trials Unit, Neurobiology and Anesthesiology Branch, National Institute of Dental Research, National Institutes of Health, Bethesda, Maryland, USA*

Patricia A. McGrath, PhD, *Director, Child Health Research Institute, Associate Professor, Department of Paediatrics, The University of Western Ontario, London, Ontario, Canada*

Patrick J. McGrath, PhD, *Professor of Physiology, Pediatrics, Psychiatry, and Occupational Therapy, Dalhousie University; Pain and Palliative Care Program, IWK Children's Hospital, Halifax, Nova Scotia, Canada*

George Mendelson, MB BS, MD, FRANZCP, *Honorary Clinical Associate Professor, Department of Psychological Medicine, Monash University; Consultant Psychiatrist, Pain Management Centre, Caulfield General Medical Centre, Melbourne, Victoria, Australia*

Harold Merskey, DM, *Professor Emeritus of Psychiatry, University of Western Ontario; London Psychiatric Hospital, London, Ontario, Canada*

David Niv, MD, *Senior Lecturer in Anesthesia and Critical Care Medicine, Director, Pain Control Unit, Tel-Aviv Sourasky Medical Center; Sackler Faculty of Medicine, Tel-Aviv University, Tel Aviv, Israel*

Richard Payne, MD, *Associate Professor of Medicine (Neurology), Chief, Section of Pain and Symptom Management, Department of Neuro-Oncology, M.D. Anderson Cancer Center, Houston, Texas, USA*

Russell K. Portenoy, MD, *Director of Analgesic Studies, Pain Service, Department of Neurology, Memorial Sloan-Kettering Cancer Center; Associate Professor of Neurology, Cornell University Medical College, New York, New York, USA*

Donald D. Price, PhD, *Director of Human Research, Professor of Anesthesiology, Medical College of Virginia, Richmond, Virginia, USA*

Neil H. Raskin, MD, *Professor of Neurology, University of California, San Francisco School of Medicine, San Francisco, USA*

L. Brian Ready, MD, FRCPC, *Professor, Department of Anesthesiology, University of Washington School of Medicine; Director, University of Washington Medical Center Pain Service, Seattle, Washington, USA*

Michael C. Rowbotham, MD, *Director, UCSF Pain Clinical Research Center, Assistant Professor of Neurology and Anesthesia, University of California, San Francisco, California, USA*

John W. Scadding, BSc, MB BS, MD, FRCP, *Consultant Neurologist, The National Hospital for Neurology and Neurosurgery, Queen Square, London, United Kingdom*

Barry J. Sessle, BDS, MDS, BSc, PhD, *Dean and Professor, Faculty of Dentistry, Professor, Department of Physiology, Faculty of Medicine, University of Toronto, Toronto, Ontario, Canada*

Yair Sharav, DMD, MS, *Professor of Oral Medicine, Head, Department of Oral Diagnosis, Oral Medicine and Radiology, School of Dental Medicine, Hebrew University Hadassah, Jerusalem, Israel*

David G. Simons, MD, MS, DSc, *Clinical Professor, Department of Physical Medicine and Rehabilitation, University of California Irvine, Irvine, California, USA*

Ronald R. Tasker, MD, MA, FRCS(C), *Professor, Department of Surgery, The University of Toronto, Division of Neurosurgery, The Toronto Hospital, Western Division, Toronto, Ontario, Canada*

Dennis C. Turk, PhD, *Director, Pain Evaluation and Treatment Institute, Professor of Psychiatry, Anesthesiology, and Behavioral Science, University of Pittsburgh, Pittsburgh, Pennsylvania, USA*

Anita M. Unruh, BSc, OT, MSW, *Assistant Professor, School of Occupational Therapy, Dalhousie University, Halifax, Nova Scotia, Canada*

Sridhar V. Vasudevan, MD, FACPM, *Clinical Professor of Physical Medicine and Rehabilitation, Medical College of Wisconsin; Medical Director, Pain Rehabilitation Center, Elmbrook Memorial Hospital, Brookfield, Wisconsin, USA*

Michael Von Korff, ScD, *Associate Director for Research, Center for Health Studies, Group Health Cooperative, Seattle, Washington, USA*

George L. Wilcox, PhD, *Professor of Pharmacology, Member, Graduate Program in Neuroscience, Co-director, Center for Neuroscientific Databases, University of Minnesota Medical School, Minneapolis, Minnesota, USA*

William D. Willis, Jr., MD, PhD, *Director, Ashbel Smith Marine Biomedical Institute; Professor and Chairman of Anatomy and Neurosciences, University of Texas Medical Branch, Galveston, Texas, USA*

Clifford J. Woolf, MB BCh, PhD, MRCP, *Professor of Anatomy and Developmental Biology, University College London, London, United Kingdom*

Manfred Zimmermann, Dr-Ing, *Professor of Physiology, Head, Department of Central Nervous System Physiology, 2nd Physiological Institute, University of Heidelberg, Heidelberg, Germany*

Foreword

The last version of this curriculum was published in 1991 and, as with any evolving scholarly discipline, our knowledge base in the field of pain research and treatment has expanded at a brisk rate. The response to the first edition has been gratifying, not only because of the broad approval of the subject matter, but because it clearly has filled an important need. It has been used as a reference for other curricula, as a reference for designing training programs, as a basis for credentialing, and to help health officials rationally plan services for pain patients.

It has been very gratifying to work with my fellow professionals in developing this document. They have donated their valuable knowledge and precious time to this revision, and the result is a significantly improved curriculum. The references have been updated, many chapters expanded, and a new chapter on basic pharmacology has been added. Although we have attempted to be comprehensive, definitive, and accurate, we acknowledge that our discipline is dynamic and this document has to be considered a snapshot of a moving target. The last word is in the distant future. For an introduction to the field of pain, the task force suggests the general references listed below.

For their assistance with the production of this book, I would like to acknowledge Louisa Jones, Executive Officer of IASP; Sandy Marvinney, Production Editor; Dale Schmidt, Word Processing Technician; and Laura Harger, my assistant at the University of California, San Francisco, during initial work on this book.

HOWARD L. FIELDS, MD, PhD
Editor

General References

Aronoff, M., (Ed.), Pain Centers: Revolution in Health Care, Raven Press, New York, 1988.

Bonica, J.J., (Ed.), The Management of Pain, 2nd ed., Vol. I and II, Lea & Febiger, Philadelphia, 1990.

Cailliet, R., Pain: Mechanisms and Management, F.A. Davis, Philadelphia, 1993.

Fields, H.J., Pain, McGraw Hill, New York, 1987.

Price, D.D., Psychological and Neural Mechanisms of Pain, Raven Press, New York, 1988.

Turk, D. and Melzack, R., Handbook of Pain Assessment, Guilford Press, New York, 1992.

Wall, P.D. and R. Melzack, (Eds.), Textbook of Pain, 3rd ed., Churchill Livingstone, Edinburgh, 1994, pp. 566–573.

Willis, W.D., Jr. and Coggeshall, R.E., Sensory Mechanisms of the Spinal Cord, 2nd ed., Plenum Press, New York, 1991.

Zohn, D.A., Musculoskeletal Pain: Diagnosis and Treatment, 2nd ed., Little, Brown & Company, Boston, 1988.

Core Curriculum for Professional Education in Pain, edited by H.L. Fields, IASP Press, Seattle, © 1995.

1

Anatomy and Physiology

I. Peripheral mechanisms

    A. Know the properties of receptors supplied by cutaneous A-beta, A-delta, and C primary afferent fibers (Willis and Coggeshall 1991) and the kinds of stimuli that activate primary afferent nociceptors either directly or indirectly by producing tissue injury or inflammation. Know what distinguishes first and second pain (Lewis 1942; Treede et al. 1995). Know what approach can be used to study cutaneous nociceptors in humans (Willis and Coggeshall 1991).

    B. Be aware of how nociceptors in musculoskeletal and visceral tissues differ from cutaneous nociceptors (Ness and Gebhart 1990; Mense 1993; Schaible and Grubb 1993; Cervero 1994). Know the different qualities of pain that result from stimulation of nociceptors in deep tissue versus skin (Lewis 1942; Mense 1993).

    C. Recognize the "silent nociceptors" and the fact that these and other nociceptors can become sensitized (Handwerker and Kobal 1993; Schaible and Grubb 1993; Cervero 1994). Be aware of the sources of substances that can sensitize nociceptors, such as neurons and immune cells (Dray 1994). Understand that second-messenger systems have a role in the sensitization of nociceptors (Taiwo et al. 1990; Dray 1994). Know the role of eicosanoids and cyclooxygenase in nociception (Mense 1993; Schaible and Grubb 1993; Dray 1994), and be aware that there may be other mechanisms of analgesic action of nonsteroidal anti-inflammatory drugs (NSAIDs) than inhibition of cyclooxygenase (McCormack 1994).

    D. Know the characteristics of neurogenic inflammation (Lewis 1942; Dray 1994). Be aware of the efferent functions of primary afferent fibers and the consequences of antidromic activation of primary afferent nociceptors, by either axon reflexes or dorsal root reflexes (Holzer 1988; Sluka et al. 1995). Know what primary hyperalgesia is and what might cause it (Lewis 1942; Hardy 1952; Willis 1992). Know how primary hyperalgesia differs from allodynia and secondary hyperalgesia.

    E. Know what peptides are found in primary afferent nociceptors (Willis and Coggeshall 1991). Be aware of the evidence that substance P and other neuropeptides play a role both in nociception and in neurogenic inflammation (Holzer 1988; Dray 1994). Know that nonpeptide neurotransmitters are also used by primary afferent nociceptors (Willis and Coggeshall 1991).

    F. Be aware of the interactions between growth factors and primary afferent nociceptors (Lewin et al. 1993). Understand how the normal phenotype of primary afferent nociceptors can change during inflammation and after axotomy so that ectopic discharges and mechanical and adrenergic sensitivity can develop (Sato and Perl 1991; Kim et al. 1993; McLachlan et al. 1993; Hökfelt et al. 1994).

    G. Be aware that injury to peripheral nerves can cause central, as well as peripheral, morphological and functional changes (Dubner 1991; Snow and Wilson 1991). These changes may be responsible for peripheral and central neuropathic pain states (Bennett 1991; Woolf and Doubell 1994).

II. Central mechanisms of nociceptive transmission

   A. Know Rexed's lamination scheme for the spinal cord dorsal horn and how it relates to the marginal zone, substantia gelatinosa, and deeper layers of the dorsal horn. Know how the terminals of different types of primary afferents are distributed in the spinal cord (Willis and Coggeshall 1991).

   B. Know the response properties of different types of nociceptive neurons in the spinal cord and medullary dorsal horn, including nociceptive-specific and wide-dynamic-range neurons (Price 1988; Willis and Coggeshall 1991). Be aware of the fast and slow synaptic events that are produced by large- and small-caliber primary afferent fibers in dorsal horn neurons (Thompson et al. 1993). Know the neurotransmitters and receptor types that are involved in nociceptive signaling (Willis and Coggeshall 1991).

   C. Be aware that prolonged or repeated noxious stimuli can lower the threshold of dorsal horn neurons (sensitization) (Woolf and Doubell 1994). Know about wind-up and the afferent fibers and neurotransmitters that are responsible (Willis and Coggeshall 1991). Know that sensitization of dorsal horn neurons can be prevented or reversed by antagonists of N-methyl-D-aspartate (NMDA) and neurokinin receptors (Willis 1994).

   D. Understand that immediate early genes are expressed in dorsal horn neurons following noxious stimuli and that these transcription factors might control the expression of genes that can alter the morphology and/or function of the neurons (Zimmermann and Herdegen 1994).

   E. Understand how central sensitization might contribute to allodynia and secondary hyperalgesia (Willis 1994). What is the logical basis for preemptive analgesia (Yaksh and Abram 1993)? Be aware that nerve injury or long-term inflammation can alter sensory processing in the dorsal horn (Dubner 1991; Coderre et al. 1993). Know that nerve injury can cause large primary afferent fibers to grow into lamina II (Woolf et al. 1992).

III. Involvement of higher centers in nociceptive processing

   A. Know the central pathways and supraspinal targets of nociceptive projection neurons and evidence that can be used to implicate a neuron in nociception (Price 1988). Be aware of the thalamic nuclei and cortical areas that are involved in pain (Willis 1985; Casey 1991). Distinguish between the sensory-discriminative and motivational-affective aspects of pain and know which central nervous system structures are likely to be associated with each (Price 1988).

   B. Understand the neural basis of referred pain, including the convergence-projection theory (Willis and Coggeshall 1991). Be aware of the segmental relationship between the innervation of deep and of cutaneous tissues (Ness and Gebhart 1990). Know what a projected sensation is. Know that nociceptive inputs can cause flexion reflexes and also changes in the sympathetic output, and the theory that these somatic and autonomic reflexes can amplify and prolong pain (Mense 1993).

IV. Pain modulation

   A. Understand the segmental and descending inhibitory mechanisms that affect spinal nociceptive neurons (Basbaum and Fields 1978; Besson and Chaouch 1987; Fields and Besson 1988; Fields et al.1991; Light 1992; Rees and Roberts 1993; Fields and Basbaum 1994). Know the brain stem regions involved in modulation of nociceptive transmission, their interconnections, their spinal projections, and the effects of electrical or chemical stimulation.

B. Be aware of the different kinds of opioids, opioid receptors, and opioid antagonists (Lewis et al. 1987). Know the distribution of endogenous opioids and what conditions would favor their release. Know the pre- and postsynaptic distribution of opioid receptors. Distinguish between opioid analgesia and nonopioid forms of analgesia.

C. Know the distribution of serotonin- and norepinephrine-containing neurons and their brain stem and spinal cord projections and how the neurotransmitters released by these neurons in the spinal cord may be involved in modulating nociception (Besson and Chaouch 1987; Fields et al. 1991; Fields and Basbaum 1994).

D. Know the ways in which electrical stimulation can activate the endogenous analgesia system (Gybels and Sweet 1989). For instance, be aware of the experimental evidence for antinociceptive effects of peripheral nerve stimulation, dorsal column stimulation, and deep brain stimulation.

REFERENCES

The best overall references on this subject are Bonica 1990 and Wall and Melzack 1994.

Basbaum, A.I. and Fields, H.L., Endogenous pain control mechanisms: review and hypothesis, Ann. Neurol., 4 (1978) 451–462.

Bennett, G.J., Evidence from animal models on the pathogenesis of painful peripheral neuropathy: relevance for pharmacotherapy. In: A.I. Basbaum and J.M. Besson (Eds.), Towards a New Pharmacology of Pain, John Wiley & Sons, Chichester, 1991, pp. 365–379.

Besson, J.M. and Chaouch, H., Peripheral and spinal mechanisms of pain, Physiol. Rev., 67 (1987) 67–184.

Bonica, J.J. (Ed.), The Management of Pain, 2nd ed., Lea & Febiger, Philadelphia, 1990.

Casey, K.L., Pain and Central Nervous System Disease: The Central Pain Syndromes, Raven Press, New York, 1991.

Cervero, F., Sensory innervation of the viscera: peripheral basis of visceral pain, Physiol. Rev., 74 (1994) 95–138.

Coderre, T.J., Katz, J., Vaccarino, A.L. and Melzack, R., Contribution of central neuroplasticity to pathological pain: review of clinical and experimental evidence, Pain, 52 (1993) 259–285.

Dray, A., Chemical activation and sensitization of nociceptors. In: J.M. Besson, G. Guilbaud and H. Ollat (Eds.), Peripheral Neurons in Nociception: Physio-pharmacological Aspects, John Libbey Eurotext, Paris, 1994, pp. 49–70.

Dubner, R., Neuronal plasticity and pain following peripheral tissue inflammation or nerve injury. In: M.R. Bond, J.E. Charlton and C.J. Woolf (Eds.), Proceedings of the VIth World Congress on Pain, Pain Research and Clinical Management, Vol. 4, Elsevier, Amsterdam, 1991, pp. 263–276.

Fields, H.L. and Basbaum, A.I., Central nervous system mechanisms of pain modulation. In: P.D. Wall and R. Melzack (Eds.), Textbook of Pain, 3rd ed., Churchill Livingstone, Edinburgh, 1994, pp. 243–257.

Fields, H.L. and Besson, J.-M., Pain Modulation, Progress in Brain Research, Vol. 77, Elsevier, Amsterdam, 1988.

Fields, H.L., Heinricher, M.M. and Mason, P., Neurotransmitters in nociceptive modulatory circuits, Annu. Rev. Neurosci., 14 (1991) 219–245.

Gybels, J.M. and Sweet, W.H., Neurosurgical Treatment of Persistent Pain, Karger, Basel, 1989.

Handwerker, H.O. and Kobal, G., Psychophysiology of experimentally induced pain, Physiol. Rev., 73 (1993) 639–671.

Hardy, J.D., Wolff, H.G. and Goodell, H., Pain Sensations and Reactions, Hafner Publishing Co., New York, 1952 [reprinted 1967].

Hökfelt, T., Zhang, X. and Wiesenfeld-Hallin, Z., Messenger plasticity in primary sensory neurons following axotomy and its functional implications, Trends Neurosci., 17 (1994) 22–30.

Holzer, P., Local effector functions of capsaicin-sensitive sensory nerve endings: involvement of tachykinins, calcitonin gene-related peptide and other neuropeptides, Neuroscience, 24 (1988) 739–768.

Kim, S.H., Heung, S.N., Kwangsup, S. and Chung, J.M., Effects of sympathectomy on a rat model of peripheral neuropathy, Pain, 55 (1993) 85–92.

Lewin, G.R., Ritter, A.M. and Mendell, L.M., Nerve growth factor-induced hyperalgesia in the neonatal and adult rat, J. Neurosci., 13 (1993) 2136–2148.

Lewis, J., Mansour, A., Khachaturian, H., Watson, S.J. and Akil, H., Opioids and pain regulation. In: H. Akil and J.W. Lewis (Eds.), Neurotransmitters and Pain Control, Karger, Basel, 1987.

Lewis, T., Pain, Macmillan, New York, 1942.

Light, A.R., The Initial Processing of Pain and Its Descending Control: Spinal and Trigeminal Systems, Karger, Basel, 1992.

McCormack, K., Non-steroidal anti-inflammatory drugs and spinal nociceptive processing, Pain, 59 (1994) 9–43.

McLachlan, E.M., Jänig, W., Devor, M. and Michaelis, M., Peripheral nerve injury triggers noradrenergic sprouting within dorsal root ganglia, Nature, 363 (1993) 543–546.

Mense, S., Nociception from skeletal muscle in relation to clinical muscle pain, Pain, 54 (1993) 241–289.

Ness, T.J. and Gebhart, G.F., Visceral pain: a review of experimental studies, Pain, 41 (1990) 167–234.

Price, D.D., Psychological and Neural Mechanisms of Pain, Raven Press, New York, 1988.

Rees, H. and Roberts, M.H.T., The anterior pretectal nucleus: a proposed role in sensory processing, Pain, 53 (1993) 121–135.

Sato, J. and Perl, E.R., Adrenergic excitation of cutaneous pain receptors induced by peripheral nerve injury, Science, 251 (1991) 1608–1610.

Schaible, H.-G. and Grubb, B.D., Afferent and spinal mechanisms of joint pain, Pain, 55 (1993) 5–54.

Sluka, K.A., Willis, W.D. and Westlund, K.N., The role of dorsal root reflexes in neurogenic inflammation, Pain Forum, 4 (1995) 141–149.

Snow, P.J. and Wilson, P., Plasticity in the somatosensory system of developing and mature mammals: the effects of injury to the central and peripheral nervous system. In: D. Ottoson (Ed.), Progress in Sensory Physiology, Springer-Verlag, Berlin, 1991.

Taiwo, Y.O., Bjerknes, L.K., Goetzl, E.J. and Levine, J.D., Mediation of primary afferent peripheral hyperalgesia by the cAMP second messenger system, Neuroscience, 32 (1990) 577–580.

Thompson, S.W.N., Woolf, C.J. and Sivolotti, L.G., Small caliber afferents produce a heterosynaptic facilitation of the synaptic responses evoked by primary afferent A fibres in the neonatal rat spinal cord in vitro, J. Neurophysiol., 69 (1993) 2116–2128.

Treede, R.D., Meyer, R.A., Raja, S.N. and Campbell, J.N., Evidence for two different heat transduction mechanisms in nociceptive primary afferents innervating monkey skin, J. Physiol., 483 (1995) 747–758.

Wall, P.D. and Melzack, R. (Eds.), Textbook of Pain, 3rd ed., Churchill Livingstone, Edinburgh, 1994.

Willis, W.D., The Pain System: The Neural Basis of Nociceptive Transmission in the Mammalian Nervous System, Karger, Basel, 1985.

Willis, W.D. (Ed.), Hyperalgesia and Allodynia, Raven Press, New York, 1992.

Willis, W.D. Central plastic responses to pain. In: G.F. Gebhart, D.L. Hammond, and T.S. Jensen (Eds.), Proceedings of the 7th World Congress on Pain, Progress in Pain Research and Management, Vol. 2, IASP Press, Seattle, 1994, pp. 301–324.

Willis, W.D., and Coggeshall, R.E., Sensory Mechanisms of the Spinal Cord, 2nd ed., Plenum Press, New York, 1991.

Woolf, C.J. and Doubell, T.P., The pathophysiology of chronic pain: increased sensitivity to low threshold Aß-fibre inputs, Curr. Opin. Neurobiol., 4 (1994) 525–534.

Woolf, C.J., Shortland, P. and Coggeshall, R.E., Peripheral nerve injury triggers central sprouting of myelinated afferents, Nature, 355 (1992) 75–78.

Yaksh, T.L. and Abram, S.E., Preemptive analgesia: a popular misnomer, but a clinically relevant truth? APS Journal, 2 (1993) 116–121.

Zimmermann, M. and Herdegen, T., Control of gene transcription by jun and fos proteins in the nervous system: beneficial or harmful molecular mechansims of neuronal response to noxious stimulation? APS Journal, 3 (1994) 33–48.

Core Curriculum for Professional Education in Pain, edited by H.L. Fields, IASP Press, Seattle, © 1995.

2

Pharmacology of Pain Transmission and Modulation

I. Peripheral mechanisms

   A. Know that neuropeptides (e.g., substance P) and autocoids (e.g., prostaglandins) participate in peripheral events leading to hyperalgesia and edema in inflammation, including increased blood flow and promotion of hyperresponsiveness of nociceptors (Besson and Chaouch 1987; Dray and Perkins 1993; Dray et al. 1994).

   B. Be aware that other agents such as bradykinin, serotonin, histamine, and hydrogen ions (acid pH) can activate nociceptors (Dray and Perkins 1993; Dray et al. 1994).

   C. Be aware of the difference between activation and sensitization of the peripheral terminals of primary afferent nociceptors. Be aware that some compounds do both (e.g., bradykinin), whereas others are primarily sensitizing (e.g., prostaglandins).

   D. Be aware that there are several classes of anti-inflammatory agents. Be aware that cyclooxygenase, the key enzyme for the production of prostaglandins in inflammatory exudates, exists in two forms so that cyclooxygenase inhibitors with reduced gastrointestinal side effects may be possible (Dray and Perkins 1993).

   E. Know that there are cellular changes in peripheral tissues that accompany inflammation and that these may affect the responsiveness of primary afferents in both a positive and negative direction (e.g., appearance of opioid-releasing immune cells) (Hargreaves 1993). Know that populations of silent nociceptors may become active during inflammation.

   F. Be aware that there are growth factors, nerve growth factor (NGF) for example, that are produced by neural and nonneural tissue and that may influence responsiveness and regrowth of damaged neural tissue (McMahon et al. 1993; Dray et al. 1994).

   G. Know the basis for sympathetic influences on pain (Chapters 9 and 19, this volume).

II. Synaptic transmission in dorsal horn

   A. Know that glutamate is an excitatory amino acid (EAA) implicated in transmission from primary afferent nociceptors to dorsal horn neurons. Be aware that there are several types of EAA receptors and that various combinations of these subtypes exist on dorsal horn neurons and determine the time course of their response to noxious stimuli and their different susceptibilities to pharmacological agents (Wilcox 1991a; Dickenson 1994b; Dray et al. 1994).

   B. Understand the processes that underlie wind-up and central hyperalgesia. Be aware of the postulated role of N-methyl-D-aspartate (NMDA) type of EAA receptor in these processes. Know that ketamine and dextromethorphan block the NMDA receptor complex (Dickenson 1994b; Price et al. 1994).

C. Know that some neuropeptides present in primary afferent nociceptors are excitatory (e.g., including substance P and CGRP (calcitonin-gene-related peptide) while others are inhibitory (e.g., somato-statin) to dorsal horn neurons.

D. Understand the importance of modulation of transmitter release from nerve terminals through such mechanisms as reduction of Ca^{++} influx, hyperpolarization, and alteration of levels of intracellular second messengers (Dickenson 1994b; Price et al. 1994).

E. Understand the importance of postsynaptic modulation of transmission (Fields et al. 1991).

F. Be aware that prostaglandins, which result from cyclooxygenase activity, are present in and affect synaptic transmission in the spinal cord as well as contribute to inflammatory pain in peripheral tissues; therefore, cyclooxygenase inhibitors such as aspirin and NSAIDs may have both peripheral and central nervous system (CNS) actions relevant to analgesia (Yaksh and Malmberg 1994).

III. Central sensitization

A. Know the physiological characteristics of the afferent input required to initiate the glutamate-receptor-mediated prolonged enhancement of excitatory synaptic transmission to dorsal horn nociceptive neurons (i.e., prolonged burst in unmyelinated primary afferent input) (Wilcox 1991a ; McMahon et al. 1993; Dickenson 1994b; Dray et al. 1994).

B. Know the broad classes of agents capable of blocking the development of central sensitization (McQuay and Dickenson 1990; Wilcox 1991a; McMahon et al. 1993; Dickenson 1994b).

C. Be aware that central sensitization is more susceptible to inhibitory or analgesic agents when they are administered before rather than after the initiating afferent barrage. Know that this is the rationale used to justify preemptive analgesia (McQuay and Dickenson 1990; Coderre et al. 1993; Dickenson 1994b; Woolf 1994).

D. Be aware that central sensitization has been observed in laboratory models of neuropathic pain (Woolf and Doubell 1994).

E. Know that pain-signaling transmitters can activate the expression of certain genes and the production of highly diffusible mediators such as the gas nitric oxide (NO). These changes may contribute to central sensitization (Dubner and Ruda 1992; Meller and Gebhart 1993; Dray et al. 1994).

F. Be aware of the possible sites of action of anticonvulsants and excitability blockers at both central and peripheral sites (Dray et al. 1994).

IV. Neurotransmitters in pain modulation

A. Know the broad array of receptor systems that couple transmitter and analgesic drug action to analgesic effects (Yaksh and Noueihed 1985; Wilcox 1993; Dickenson 1994a).

B. Know the three main types of opioid receptors and the variations in effectiveness of drugs acting on each type (Yaksh and Noueihed 1985; Wilcox 1993; Dickenson 1994a). Be aware that cloning of the opioid receptors has led to detailed knowledge of their structure and, through antibodies, to their precise location in the brain (Dickenson 1994a; Uhl et al. 1994).

C. Understand that numerous factors, such as nerve injury and inflammation, can reduce and enhance opioid analgesia (Chapter 7, this volume; Dickenson 1994). Be aware of proposed mechanisms of opioid tolerance (Wilcox 1993; Basbaum 1995).

D. Know that opioid agonists act in the central nervous system at both spinal and supraspinal sites involved in pain transmission and modulation (Yaksh and Noueihed 1985; Besson and Chaouch 1987; Meller and Gebhart 1993).

E. Be aware that several neurotransmitters are involved in descending pain modulation from brainstem analgesic centers (e.g., norepinephrine, serotonin, glutamate, and GABA) (Yaksh and Noueihed 1985; Besson and Chaouch 1987; Fields et al. 1991; Dickenson 1994a). Understand that these neurotransmitters bind to different receptor classes so that some neurotransmitters interact synergistically and others will interact antagonistically (Dickenson and Sullivan 1993). Understand the use of adjuncts of enhance opioid analgesia (Dickenson and Sullivan 1993; Dickenson 1994a; Yaksh and Malmberg 1994).

REFERENCES

Basbaum, A.I., Insights into the development of opioid tolerance, Pain, 61 (1995) 349–352.

Besson, J.-M, and Chaouch, A., Peripheral and spinal mechanisms of nociception, Physiol. Rev., 67 (1987) 67–186.

Coderre, T.J., Katz, J., Vaccarino, A.L. and Melzack, R., Contribution of central neuroplasticity to pathological pain: review of clinical and experimental evidence, Pain, 52 (1993) 259–285.

Devor, M., Wall, P.D. and Catalan, N., Systemic lidocaine silences ectopic neuroma and DRG discharge without blocking nerve conduction, Pain, 48 (1992) 261–268.

Dickenson, A.H., Where and how opioids act. In: G.F. Gebhart, D.L. Hammond and T. Jensen, (Eds.), Proceedings of the 7th World Congress on Pain, Progress in Pain Research and Management, Vol. 2., IASP Press, Seattle, 1994a, pp. 525–552.

Dickenson, A.H., NMDA receptor antagonists as analgesics. In: H.L. Fields and J.C. Liebeskind (Eds.), Pharmacological Approaches to the Treatment of Pain: New Concepts and Critical Issues, Progress in Pain Research and Management, Vol. 1, IASP Press, Seattle, 1994b, pp. 173–187.

Dickenson, A.H. and Sullivan, A.F., Combination therapy in analgesia: seeking synergy, Current Opinion in Anaesthesiology, 6 (1993) 861–865.

Dray, A. and Perkins, M.N., Bradykinin and inflammatory pain, Trends Neurosci., 16 (1993) 99–104.

Dray, A., Urban, L. and Dickenson, A.H., Pharmacology of chronic pain, Trends Pharmacol. Sci., 15 (1994) 190–197.

Dubner, R. and Ruda, M.A., Activity-dependent neuronal plasticity following tissue injury and inflammation, Trends Neurosci., 15 (1992) 96–103.

Fields, H.L., Heinricher, M.M. and Mason, P., Neurotransmitters in nociceptive modulatory circuits, Annu. Rev. Neurosci., 14 (1991) 219–245.

Hargreaves, L., Peripheral opioid analgesia, APS Journal, 2 (1993) 50–55.

McMahon, S.B., Lewin, G.R. and Wall, P.D., Central excitability triggered by noxious inputs, Curr. Opin. Neurobiol., 3 (1993) 602–610.

McQuay, H. and Dickenson, A.H., Implications of central nervous system plasticity for pain management, Anaesthesiology, 45 (1990) 101–102

Meller, S.T. and Gebhart, G.F., Nitric oxide (NO) and nociceptive processing in the spinal cord, Pain, 52 (1993) 127–136.

Price, D.D., Mao, J. and Mayer, D.J., Central neural mechanisms of normal and abnormal pain states. In: H.L. Fields and J.C. Liebeskind (Eds.), Pharmacological Approaches to the Treatment of Pain: New Concepts and Critical Issues, Progress in Pain Research and Management, Vol. 1, IASP Press, Seattle, 1994, pp. 61–84.

Uhl, G.R., Childers, S. and Pasternak, G., An opiate receptor gene family reunion, Trends Neurosci., 17 (1994) 89–93.

Wilcox, G.L., Excitatory neurotransmitters and pain. In: M. Bond, C.J. Woolf and J.E. Charlton (Eds.), Proceedings of the VIth World Congress on Pain, Pain Research and Clinical Management, Elsevier Science Publishers BV, Amsterdam, 1991, pp. 97–117.

Wilcox, G.L., Sources and cellular targets for peripherally acting analgesics mediated by G protein-coupled receptors, APS Journal, 2 (1993a) 60–65.

Wilcox, G.L. Spinal modulators of nociceptive neurotransmission and hyperalgesia: relationships among synaptic plasticity, analgesic tolerance and blood flow, APS Journal, 2 (1993b) 265–275.

Woolf, C.J., A new strategy for the treament of inflammatory pain, Drugs, suppl. 5 (1994) 1–9.

Woolf, C.J. and Doubell, T.P., The pathophysiology of chronic pain: increased sensitivity to low-threshold $\alpha\beta$-fibre inputs, Curr. Opin. Neurobiol., 4 (1994) 525–534.

Yaksh, T.L. and Noueihed, R., The physiology and pharmacology of spinal opiates, Annu. Rev. Pharmacol. Toxicol., 25 (1985) 433–462.

Yaksh, T.L. and Malmberg, A.B., Interaction of spinal modulatory systems. In: H.L. Fields and J.C. Liebeskind (Eds.), Pharmacological Approaches to the Treatment of Pain: New Concepts and Critical Issues, Progress in Pain Research Management, Vol. 1, IASP Press, Seattle, 1994, pp. 151–171.

Core Curriculum for Professional Education in Pain, edited by H.L. Fields, IASP Press, Seattle, © 1995.

3

Pain Measurement in Humans

I. Understand the basic concepts in pain measurement (Turk and Melzack 1992).

   A. Pain is conceptualized as a human experience and is primarily measured by subjective report (Price and Harkins 1992; Gracely 1994).

   B. Understand current models of pain, which characterize it as having sensory, cognitive, and motivational-affective dimensions (Sternbach 1986; Osterweis et al. 1987; Gracely 1992, 1994; Price and Harkins 1992).

   C. Understand the differences between acute, chronic, and recurrent pain.

   D. Comprehend the difference between pain measurement and pain complaint.

   E. Understand the concept of disability in relation to pain (Osterweis et al. 1987; Chapman and Loeser 1990; Tait et al. 1990).

   F. Know the meaning of reliability and validity and their importance for pain measurement (Chapman and Loeser 1990; Gracely 1992, 1994).

   G. Differentiate between concepts of nociception, pain, pain behaviors, and the emotional manifestations of pain (Chapman and Loeser 1990).

II. Understand the role of pain measurement in clinical activity, clinical research, and medical-legal determinations (Max et al. 1990; Dirks et al. 1993; Gracely et al., in press).

   A. Be able to interpret pain measurement for diagnosis (Grossman 1994; Gracely et al., in press).

   B. Be able to quantify pain when evaluating treatment effect (Max et al. 1990).

   C. Comprehend the importance of measurement in research on pain control (Chapman and Loeser 1990).

   D. Understand the place of pain assessment scores in postoperative and other patient charts (Faries 1991).

   E. Understand issues in the assessment of pain disability (Follick et al. 1986; Osterweis et al. 1987).

III. Understand basic approaches to measuring pain.

   A. Be able to use subjective report methods and understand the advantages and limitations of each method (Gracely 1994; Jensen et al. 1986).

1. Understand the following simple tools:

    a. Verbal category scale (Jensen et al. 1986; Gracely 1992, 1994)
    b. Numerical category or rating scale (Jensen et al. 1986; Gracely 1992, 1994)
    c. Visual analog scale (Price et al. 1994; Turk and Melzack 1992)
    d. Magnitude estimation and cross-modality matching (Gracely 1992, 1994)
    e. Verbal descriptor scales (Gracely 1992, 1994)

2. Understand the basic principles of one or more complex, multidimensional tools such as the McGill Pain Questionnaire and Brief Pain Inventory (Turk and Melzack 1992; Von-Korff et al. 1992; Dirks et al. 1993, Cleeland and Ryan 1994).

3. Understand the principles and methods of measuring pain in children and neonates (Bozzette 1993; Craig et al. 1993; McGrath and Unruh 1994).

    a. Behavioral rating scales
    b. Developmentally sensitive self-report scales
    c. Methods of evaluating pain expression (Craig et al. 1993; McGrath and Unruh 1994)

4. Know the basic issues and problems of assessing pain in the elderly (Harkins et al. 1994).

B. Be able to use behavioral observation methods and understand the advantages and limitations of each method (Chapman and Loeser 1990; Keefe et al. 1990; Broome 1991; Anderson et al. 1992).

    1. Understand the concept of pain behavior.
    2. Be able to design simple pain behavior ratings that can be used by staff (Broome 1991).
    3. Understand the concept of scoring complex behavior patterns.

C. Be able to use pain activity questionnaires (Baillie 1993).

    1. Understand the concept of a pain and activity diary, up-time, and down-time.
    2. Be aware of the existence of complex formal inventories relating activities to pain report.
    3. Know the limitations of this class of measurement tool.

D. Know the advantages and limitations of physiological measures (Chapman and Loeser 1990).

E. Quantitative sensory testing: measuring evoked pain in patients (Gracely et al., in press).

F. Be aware of methods and issues in the assessment of a pain-control intervention.

IV. Be able to assess factors that can bias pain measurement (White et al. 1985; Osterweis et al. 1987; Gracely 1994; Price et al., in press).

A. Comprehend the potential influence of both the immediate and the home environment on the pain report.

B. Understand how the patient's beliefs or expectations in a given circumstance can influence the pain report (Price et al., in press).

C. Understand how the clinician's beliefs or expectations can influence a patient's pain report (Gracely et al. 1985).

D. Understand the potential influence of affect disturbances and limited coping skills on the pain report.

E. Be alert to the possible influence of cultural background, age, and gender roles on the pain report.

F. Understand the concept of suffering and the possible influence of suffering on the pain report.

G. Understand the concept of the placebo effect and the problems of identifying potential placebo responses (White et al. 1985; Price et al., in press).

V. Know what makes good clinical pain measurement (Chapman and Loeser 1990; Turk and Melzack 1992; Gracely 1994).

A. Understand why more than one measurement should be used.

B. Appreciate the importance of the instruments fitting both the patient and the setting.

C. Have a grasp of quality control in pain measurement and be able to understand the importance of:

1. Patient cooperation
2. How missing data are handled (Little and Rubin 1987)
3. The measurement circumstances

   a. Patient's medications at time of measurement
   b. Presence of spouse or other influence
   c. Whether the patient has more than one pain

D. Know the burden imposed on the responder by the pain measurement tools used and how to minimize this burden.

REFERENCES

Anderson, K.O., Bradley, L.A., Turner, R.A., Agudelo, C.A., Pisko, E.J., Salley, A.N., Jr. and Fletcher, K.E., Observation of pain behavior in rheumatoid arthritis patients' physical examination: relationship to disease activity and psychological variables, Arthritis Care Research, 5(1) (1992) 49–56.

Baillie, L., A review of pain assessment tools, Nursing Standards, 7(23) (1993) 25–29.

Bozzette, M., Observation of pain behavior in the NICU: an exploratory study, Journal of Perinatal and Neonatal Nursing, 7(1) (1993) 76–87.

Broome, M.E., Measurement of behavioral response to pain, J. Pediatr. Oncol. Nurs., 8 (1991) 180–182.

Chapman, C.R. and Loeser, J.D. (Eds.), Issues in Pain Measurement, Raven Press, New York, 1990.

Cleeland, C.S. and Ryan, K.M., Pain assessment: global use of the Brief Pain Inventory, Ann. Acad. Med. Singapore, 23 (1994) 129–138.

Craig, K.D., Whitfield, M.F., Grunau, R.V., Linton, J. and Hadjistavropoulos, H.D., Pain in the preterm neonate: behavioural and physiological indices, Pain, 52 (1993) 287–299, see also erratum, Pain, 54 (1993) 111.

Dirks, J.F., Wunder, J., Kinsman, R., McElhinny, J. and Jones, N.F., A pain rating scale and a pain behavior checklist for clinical use: development, norms, and the consistency score, Psychother. Psyschosom., 59 (1993) 41–49.

Faries, J.E., Mills, D.S., Goldsmith, K.W., Phillips, K.D. and Orr, J., Systematic pain records and their impact on pain control: a pilot study, Cancer Nurs., 14 (1991) 306–313.

Follick, M.J., Smith, T.W. and Ahern, D.K., The Sickness Impact Profile: a global measure of disability in chronic low back pain, Pain, 21 (1986) 117–126.

Gracely, R.H., Evaluation of multidimensional pain scales, Pain, 48 (1992) 297–300.

Gracely, R.H., Studies of pain in normal man. In: P.D. Wall and R. Melzack (Eds.), Textbook of Pain, 3rd ed., Churchill Livingstone, London, 1994, pp. 303–313.

Gracely, R.H., Dubner, R., Deeter, W.R. and Wolskee, P.J., Clinician's expectations influence placebo analgesia, Lancet I, 43 (1985) 8419.

Gracely, R.H., Price, D.D. and Bennett, G.J., Quantitative sensory testing in patients with complex regional pain syndrome I and II. In: W. Janig and M. Stanton-Hicks (Eds.), Reflex Sympa thetic Dystrophy: A Reappraisal, Progress in Pain Research and Management, Vol. 6, IASP Press, Seattle, in press.

Grossman, S.A., Assessment of cancer pain: a continuous challenge, Support. Care Cancer, 2 (1994) 105–110.

Harkins, S.W., Price, D.D., Bush, F.M. and Small, R., Geriatric pain. In: P.D. Wall and R. Melzack (Eds.), Textbook of Pain, 3rd ed., Churchill Livingstone, London, 1994, pp 769–786.

Jensen, M.P., Karoly, P. and Braver, S., The measurement of clinical pain intensity: a comparison of six methods, Pain, 27 (1986) 117–126.

Keefe, F.J., Bradley, L.A. and Crisson, J.E., Behavioral assessment of low back pain: identification of pain behavior subgroups, Pain, 2 (1990) 153–160.

Little, R.J.A. and Rubin, D.B., Statistical Analysis with Missing Data, John Wiley & Sons, New York, 1987.

Max, M.B., Portenoy, R.K. and Laska, E.M. (Eds.), The Design of Clinical Analgesic Trials, Raven Press, New York, 1990.

McGrath, P.J. and Unruh, A.M., Measurement and assessment of paediatric pain. In: P.D. Wall and R. Melzack (Eds.), Textbook of Pain, 3rd ed., Churchill Livingstone, London, 1994, pp. 1297–1308.

Osterweis, M., Kleinman, A. and Mechanic, D., Pain and Disability: Clinical, Behavioral and Policy Perspectives, National Academy Press, Washington, DC, 1987.

Price, D.D. and Harkins, S.W., The affective-motivational dimension of pain: a two-stage model, APS Journal, 1 (1992) 229–239.

Price, D.D., Bush, F.M., Long, S. and Harkins, S.W., A comparison of pain measurement characteristics of mechanical visual analogue scales and simple numerical rating scales, Pain, 56 (1994) 217–226.

Price, D.D., Gracely, R.H. and Bennett, G.J., The challenge and the problem of placebo in assessment of sympathetically maintained pain. In: W. Janig and M. Stanton-Hicks (Eds.), Reflex Sympathetic Dystrophy: A Reappraisal, Progress in Pain Research and Management, Vol. 6, IASP Press, Seattle, in press.

Sternbach, R.A., Clinical aspects of pain. In: The Psychology of Pain, 2nd ed., Raven Press, New York, 1986, pp. 223–239.

Tait, R.C., Chibnall, J.T. and Krause, S., The Pain Disability Index: psychometric properties, Pain, 40 (1990) 171–182.

Turk, D.C. and Melzack, R. (Eds.), Handbook of Pain Assessment, Guilford Press, New York, 1992.

Von-Korff, M., Ormel, J., Keefe, F.J. and Dworkin, S.F., Grading the severity of chronic pain, Pain, 50 (1992) 133–149.

White, L., Turskey, M.B. and Schwartz, G.E., Placebo: Theory, Research, and Mechanisms, Guilford Press, New York, 1985.

Wiener, S.L., Differential Diagnosis of Acute Pain by Body Region, McGraw-Hill, Inc., New York, 1993.

Williams, R.C., Towards a set of reliable and valid measures for chronic pain assessment and outcome research, Pain, 35 (1988) 239–254.

Core Curriculum for Professional Education in Pain, edited by H.L. Fields, IASP Press, Seattle, © 1995.

4

Psychosocial Aspects of Pain

I. Definition and measurement of pain (Turk and Melzack 1992; Merskey and Bogduk 1994)

   A. Know the definition of pain as a biopsychosocial experience. Know that pain is a subjective experience with important affective, cognitive, and behavioral as well as sensory components (Turk et al. 1983; Osterweis et al. 1987; Merskey and Bogduk 1994).

   B. Recognize that pain is experienced in an emotional, cognitive, and socioenvironmental context (Turk et al. 1983).

   C. Know that pain measurement is fundamentally inferential. Thus, although the objective is to understand the subjective experience, this can be accomplished only through the interpretation of the verbal (self-report) and nonverbal behavior of the person (Turk and Melzack 1992).

   D. Distinguish between pain as a subjective experience, pain behavior as a pattern of audible or observable actions (e.g., posture, facial expression, verbalizations), and disability associated with physical and emotional functioning in all areas of life activities (Turk et al. 1983; Hadjistavropoulos and Craig 1994).

   E. Distinguish the major psychological and behavioral consequences of acute and chronic pain. For chronic pain, distinguish the major psychological components of reactions to intermittent, continuous, and progressive pain, and pain syndromes associated with terminal illness (Turk et al. 1983; Hadjistavropoulos and Craig 1994).

   F. Recognize that verbal reports provide unique access to subjective experiences, but have limitations, including response biases, and are complemented by nonverbal behavior (Prkachin and Craig 1995). Also, recognize that nonverbal behavior must be interpreted by the observer, and the inferences of the observer can be erroneous or biased (Turk and Flor 1987).

   G. Be familiar with the psychometric concepts of reliability, validity, utility, standardization, and norms. Understand that many psychological tests have not been standardized or validated on pain populations and thus extrapolation may be inappropriate, leading to invalid conclusions (Turk 1990).

II. Individual differences (Pennebaker 1982; Pilowksy 1990)

   A. Recognize the substantial variability in response to actual tissue damage, potential tissue damage, or stress as reflected in the modest correlations among physical impairment, pain, and disability (Waddell et al. 1980; Sternbach 1986; Osterweis et al. 1987).

   B. Understand the concepts of state and trait as measured by psychological tests. Be aware that trait characteristics over time may be changed by the chronic pain state, so that the psychological profile may become emotionally disturbed (e.g., depressed, anxious) (Naliboff et al. 1988; Hadjistavropoulos and Craig 1994).

C. Recognize individual differences in affective, cognitive, and behavioral responses to pain.

1. Affective processes (Fernandez and Turk 1992; Craig 1994; Hadjistavropoulos and Craig 1994)

    a. Understand the various emotional reactions to actual or potential tissue damage, including anxiety, depression, and anger.
    b. Distinguish affective states associated with acute, recurrent, and chronic pain.
    c. Know that anticipatory anxiety and fear during the pain experience may accelerate the severity of distress, or in unusual circumstances reduce distress.

2. Cognitive processes (Pennebaker 1982; Van Dalfsen and Syrjala 1989; Jensen et al. 1991; Turk and Rudy 1992)

    a. Be able to describe basic cognitive processes that determine the nature of painful experiences, including attention, expectancy, cognitive appraisals, cognitive strategies, somatic preoccupation, labeling, observational learning memory, and beliefs (Turk and Rudy 1992).
    b. Describe the major cognitive coping strategies that may enhance pain endurance or facilitate distress (i.e., attention diversion, imagery, fantasy, or redefinitions) (Fernandez and Turk 1989). Appreciate the potential ineffectiveness of passive strategies such as praying or hoping (Keefe et al. 1992).
    c. Describe the major interactions between cognitive appraisals and affective reactions (e.g., the role of catastrophizing and other maladaptive patterns of thinking, the consequences of perceived self-efficacy, personal control, and convictions of helplessness and hopelessness (Jensen et al. 1991; Turk and Rudy 1992).
    d. Distinguish the coping strategies for acute pain (e.g., trauma, postoperative) and chronic pain (e.g., low back, cancer) (Cleeland and Tearman 1986).

3. Behavioral processes (Fordyce 1976; Keefe and Gil 1986)

    a. Understand the principles of operant theory as they relate to the acquisition and maintenance of pain behavior and their role in devising intervention strategies (i.e., primary and secondary reinforcement, punishment, extinction, schedules of reinforcement, shaping, avoidance learning, stimulus control, modeling and observational learning).
    b. Know the distinction between operant and respondent conditioning (Fordyce 1976).
    c. Describe the major behavioral treatment strategies in controlling medication abuse, exercise and fitness, pain and well behavior, and disability (e.g., positive reinforcement, extinction, relaxation, biofeedback, goal setting) (Gatchel and Turk 1995).

4. Be familiar with how each of the factors described in 1–3 affects compliance with treatment recommendations and relapse following initially successful treatment (Turk and Rudy 1991).

5. Origins of individual differences (Craig 1986)

    a. Describe the major developmental changes in pain perception from birth through mature adulthood to old age (McGrath 1990; Roy 1995).
    b. Describe the process whereby socialization within the family and society, through direct experience, instruction, modeling and observational learning, and reinforcement of sanctioned behavior, leads to variations in pain and illness behavior and sick roles.

     c. Recognize that life experiences can equip a person with substantial resiliency and effective coping skills.

III. Emotional problems and psychiatric disorders associated with pain

    A. With regard to the relationship of pain and depression:

       1. Be aware of the uncertainty of establishing that depression, as a state or disorder, or any psychiatric disorder, predisposes a person to the development of a chronic pain syndrome, results in a more chronic condition, or develops as a consequence of chronic pain (Dworkin and Cligor 1988). Know that chronic pain is *not* masked depression, nor is there any evidence for the concept of a pain-prone disorder.

       2. Be aware that emotional disturbance in chronic pain patients is more likely to be a consequence than a cause of chronic pain; but that psychological events may be risk factors for the development of chronic pain (Gamsa 1990). In addition, the development of emotional disturbance may be modulated by the severity of the chronic pain at that time.

       3. Understand that the states of depression seen in psychiatric patients often differ from those of chronic pain patients. In chronic pain states both depression and pain tend to be chronic (Dworkin and Cligor 1988).

       4. Understand that the presence of depression may be a predictor of severity of pain behavior (Craig 1994).

    B. Understand the complex interaction of pain expression with the following psychological factors:

       1. Understand that personality disorders (American Psychiatric Association 1994) and maladaptive coping styles are frequently found in chronic pain patients, but it is not known whether the prevalence of personality disorders or certain subtypes of personality disorders is greater in chronic pain patients than in the general population (Fishbain et al. 1986; Fishbain et al. 1989; American Psychiatric Association 1994).

       2. Understand that chronic pain is a severe stressor that affects all aspects of a person's life— vocational, social, familial, financial, recreational, and physical. Be aware that a chronic pain state itself creates additional stressors and problems (e.g., financial, family functioning, work functioning, social, legal) (Turk et al. 1983).

       3. Understand that persons who are vulnerable to stress may perceive acute or chronic pain as catastrophic. Such vulnerabilities appear in certain personality disorders and in people who are prone to develop psychiatric symptoms under stress (e.g., those who are habitually anxious, oversensitive, obsessional, somatically preoccupied, paranoid, depressive, irritable) (Sternbach 1986).

       4. Be aware that in the psychiatric hospital and clinic populations, the complaint of pain is generally associated with anxiety, depression, and somatoform disorders (Fishbain et al. 1986).

       5. Understand the DSM-IV concepts of somatoform disorders (somatization, conversion, pain hypochondriasis, body dysmorphic disorders, factitious disorders, and malingering) (American Psychiatric Association 1994; Lipowski 1988).

       6. Be aware that chronic pain patients can present with signs and symptoms that are incongruent with medical expectations based upon anatomic and physiologic knowledge (e.g., Waddell's nonorganic signs and symptoms; Waddell et al. 1980). Appreciate that they are related to emotional distress and cognitive dysfunction, that they are not associated with malingering, and that they predict limited success with conventional medical treatment, but their reliability and validity in psychiatric diagnosis is controversial (Waddell et al. 1989; Hadjistavropoulos and Craig 1994).

C. Understand the distinction between the terms drug abuse, addiction, physical dependence, psychological dependence, and tolerance and how these concepts apply to chronic pain patients (Fishbain et al. 1992).

IV. Sociocultural variation (Koopman et al. 1984; Craig 1986; Bates 1987)

A. Know that pain behaviors and complaints are best understood in the context of social transactions among the individual, family, employers, health professionals, community, governmental agencies, and others.

B. Recognize that social factors, including beliefs about the origins and nature of pain and how one should access health care, influence both experiential and expressive features of pain.

C. Know that there are cultural variations in pain experience and expression.

D. Describe how health care professionals should be responsive to cultural variations when assessing and managing pain.

E. Understand that the workplace and the employee's appraisal of the work environment are potential sources of variation in pain, illness behavior, and disability.

F. Recognize people's sensitivity to the pain experience of others.

G. Be aware that people will vary in how they respond to the suffering of others.

V. Situational and environmental factors (Craig 1986)

A. Appreciate the propensity of a person to try to maximize access to the best treatment by influencing those perceived to be in positions of authority.

B. Recognize that others who display adaptive or excessive pain behavior can influence how patients express pain.

C. Appreciate that communications of pain, distress, and suffering by patients can elicit responses from health care providers and significant others.

D. Know the capacity of health care professionals to instigate maladaptive or adaptive reactions.

VI. The family and pain (Craig 1986; Turk et al. 1987; Rowat et al. 1994)

A. Be aware of the significance of family stress and discord as predisposing, exacerbating, or maintaining factors in pain complaints and disability.

B. Describe the potential role of the family for promoting illness or well behavior.

C. Describe the role of familial models of pain complaint and disability as predisposing factors toward maladaptive responses and disability.

D. Recognize the role of family trauma (e.g., marital discord, family violence) in increasing vulnerability to chronic pain as well as exacerbating or maintaining maladaptive behavioral responses and disability.

E. Be aware of the consequences for the family of a member suffering from chronic pain.

REFERENCES

American Psychiatric Association staff, Diagnostic and Statistical Manual of Mental Disorders: DSM-IV, American Psychiatric Association, Washington, DC, 1994.

Bates, M.S., Ethnicity and pain: a biocultural model, Soc. Sci. Med., 24 (1987) 47–50.

Cleeland, C.S. and Tearman, B.H., Behavioral control of cancer pain. In: A.D. Holzman and D.C. Turk (Eds.), Pain Management: A Handbook of Psychological Treatment Approaches, Pergamon Press, New York, 1986, pp. 193–212.

Craig, K.D., Social modeling influences: pain in context. In: R.A. Sternbach (Ed.), The Psychology of Pain, 2nd ed., Raven Press, New York, 1986, pp 67–96.

Craig, K.D., Emotional aspects of pain. In: P.D. Wall and R. Melzack (Eds.), Textbook of Pain, 3rd ed., Churchill Livingstone, Edinburgh, 1994, pp. 261–274.

Dworkin, R.H. and Cligor, E., Psychiatric diagnosis and chronic pain: DSM-III-R and beyond, J. Pain Symptom Manage., 3 (1988) 87–98.

Fernandez, E. and Turk, D.C., The utility of cognitive coping strategies for altering pain perception, Pain, 38 (1989) 125–135.

Fernandez, E. and Turk, D.C., Nociception and emotion: separation and synthesis, Psychol. Bull., 112 (1992) 205–217.

Fishbain, D.A., Goldberg, M. and Meagher, R., Male and female chronic pain patients categorized by DSM-III psychiatric diagnostic criteria, Pain, 26 (1986) 181–197.

Fishbain, D.A., Goldberg, M., Steele, R. and Rosomoff, H., DSM-III diagnoses of patients with myofascial pain syndrome (fibrositis), Arch. Phys. Med. Rehabil., 70 (1989) 433–438.

Fishbain, D.A., Rosomoff, H.L. and Rosomoff, R.S., Drug abuse, dependence, and addiction in chronic pain patients, Clin. J. Pain, 8 (1992) 77–85.

Fordyce, W.E., Behavioral Methods in Chronic Pain and Illness, C.V. Mosby, St. Louis, 1976.

Hadjistavropoulos, H.D. and Craig, K.D., Acute and chronic low back pain: cognitive, affective, and behavioral dimensions, J. Consult. Clin. Psychol., 62 (1994) 341–349.

Gamsa, A., Is emotional disturbance a precipitator or a consequence of chronic pain? Pain, 42 (1990) 183–195.

Gatchel, R.J. and Turk, D.C., Psychological Approaches to Pain Management: A Practitioner's Handbook, Guilford Press, New York, 1995.

Jensen, M.P., Turner, J.A., Romano, J.M. and Karoly, P., Coping with pain: a critical review of the literature, Pain, 47 (1991) 249–284.

Keefe, F.J. and Gil, K.M., Behavioral concepts in the analysis of chronic pain syndromes, J. Consult. Clin. Psychol., 54 (1986) 776–783.

Keefe, F.J., Salley, A.N., Jr. and Lefebvre, J.C., Coping with pain: conceptual concerns and future directions, Pain, 51 (1992) 131–134.

Koopman, S., Eisenthal, S. and Stoeckle, J., Ethnicity in the reported pain syndromes, Soc. Sci. Med., 19 (1984) 1279–1298.

Lipowski, Z.J., Somatization: the concept and its clinical application, Am. J. Psychiatry, 145 (1988) 1358–1368.

McGrath, P.A., Pain in Children. Nature, Assessment, and Treatment, Guilford Press, New York, 1990.

Merskey, H. and Bogduk, N. (Eds.), Classification of Chronic Pain: Descriptions of Chronic Pain Syndromes and Definition of Pain Terms, 2nd ed., IASP Press, Seattle, 1994.

Naliboff, B.D., McCreary, C.P., McArthur, D.L., Cohen, M.J. and Gottlieb, H.J., MMPI changes following behavioral treatment of chronic low back pain, Pain, 35 (1988) 271–277.

Osterweis, M., Kleinman, A. and Mechanic, D., Pain and Disability: Clinical, Behavioral and Policy Perspective, National Academy Press, Washington, 1987.

Pennebaker, J.W., The Psychology of Physical Symptoms, Springer-Verlag, New York, 1982.

Pilowksy, I., The concept of abnormal illness behavior, Psychosomatics, 31 (1990) 207–213.

Prkachin, K.M. and Craig, K.D., Expressing pain: the communication and interpretation of facial pain signals, J. Nonverb. Behav., in press.

Rowat, K.M., Jeans, M.E. and LeFort, S.M., A collaborative model of care: patient, family and health professionals. In: P.D. Wall and R. Melzack (Eds.), Textbook of Pain, 3rd ed., Churchill Livingstone, Edinburgh, 1994, pp. 1381–1386.

Roy, R. (Ed.), Chronic Pain in Old Age. An Integrated Biopsychosocial Perspective, University of Toronto Press, Toronto, 1995.

Sternbach, R.A., Clinical aspects of pain. In: R.A. Sternbach (Ed.), The Psychology of Pain, 2nd ed., Raven Press, New York, 1986, pp. 223–239.

Turk, D.C., Customizing treatment for chronic pain patients: who, what and why, Clin. J. Pain, 6 (1990) 255–270.

Turk, D.C. and Flor, H., Pain greater than pain behavior: the utility and limitations of the pain behavior construct, Pain, 31 (1987) 277–295.

Turk, D.C. and Melzack, R., Handbook of Pain Assessment, Guilford Press, New York, 1992.

Turk, D.C. and Rudy, T.E., Neglected factors in chronic pain treatment outcome studies: relapse, noncompliance, and adherence enhancement, Pain, 44 (1991) 5–28.

Turk, D.C. and Rudy, T.E., Cognitive factors and persistent pain: a glimpse into Pandora's box, Cognitive Therapy and Research, 16 (1992) 99–122.

Turk, D.C., Meichenbaum, D. and Genest, M., Pain and Behavioral Medicine: A Cognitive-Behavioral Perspective, Guilford Press, New York, 1983.

Turk, D.C., Flor, H. and Rudy, T.E., Pain and families. I. Etiology, maintenance, and psychosocial impact, Pain, 30 (1987) 3–27.

Van Dalfsen, P.J. and Syrjala, K.L., Psychological strategies in acute pain management, Anesthesiology Clinics of North America, 7 (1989) 171–181.

Waddell, G., McCulloch, J.A., Kummel, E. and Venner, M., Nonorganic physical signs in low back pain, Spine, 5 (1980) 117–125.

Waddell, G., Pilowsky, I. and Bond, M.R., Clinical assessment and interpretation of illness behavior in low back pain, Pain, 39 (1989) 41–53.

Core Curriculum for Professional Education in Pain, edited by H.L Fields, IASP Press, Seattle, © 1995.

5

General Principles of Pain Evaluation and Management

I. General considerations in the evaluation of patients with pain (Fields 1987; Price 1988; Bonica 1990; McGrath 1990; Turk and Melzack 1992; Wall and Melzack 1994)

A. Know the key elements of a pain-related history and be able to use a structured interview to obtain the relevant information.

   1. Know how to assess a pain complaint with regard to the following:

      a. Temporal characteristics—mode of onset and evolution over time
      b. Location—may be determined verbally or by using a pain diagram
      c. Intensity—visual analog scales, numerical scales, or verbal scales may be used
      d. Quality—guide the patient for relevant words or use the McGill Pain Questionnaire
      e. Exacerbating and relieving factors
      f. Common validated instruments used to assess pain complaint and impact (Chapter 3)
      g. Differences between categories of pain: acute, acute treatment-related, recurrent, and persistent
      h. Evaluation of primary and secondary sources of nociceptive input

   2. Be able to obtain a history of concurrent medical illnesses that may influence the patient's pain complaints or responses to interventions.

      a. Know those medical diseases in which acute, recurrent, or chronic pain is a major component in adults and children (e.g., sickle-cell disease, cancer, and arthritis).
      b. Understand the assessment of pain in patients disabled by other diseases (with weakness, limited range of motion, or cognitive impairment).

   3. Be able to assess psychological factors and psychiatric disease as they relate to the patient's pain complaints. Understand the limitations of the medical model of disease for many patients with chronic pain and be able to assess pain in the absence of a clearly defined anatomical cause for that pain (Sternbach 1986; France and Krishnan 1988; Price 1988; American Psychiatric Association 1994; Pilowsky 1994; also see Chapter 4).

      a. Know the relationship between currently accepted DSM-IV psychiatric diagnoses (American Psychiatric Association 1994) and pain complaint. Be familiar with somatoform pain disorder, somatization disorder, depression, and hysteria. Understand how these disorders may affect the reporting of pain and how descriptors of pain relate to these diagnoses.
      b. Understand and be able to interpret the common psychological concomitants of pain (anxiety in acute pain and depression in chronic pain). Be aware of how anxiety and depression affect a pain report.
      c. Understand and be able to distinguish between normal and abnormal illness behavior. Be able to assess interpersonal factors reinforcing abnormal illness behavior.
      d. Understand the psychological issues that may be caused or altered by pain medication.

4. Understand the difference between impairment and disability. Be able to assess psychological and physical disabilities (Chapter 25).

5. Be able to take a detailed medication history.

   a. Focus on an assessment of the adequacy and unwanted actions of analgesic medications (nonsteroidal anti-inflammatory drugs and opioids) and adjuvant medications (antidepressants, anticonvulsants, and anxiolytics).
   b. Understand factors that lead to undertreatment of pain.

6. Understand pain-related issues that are unique to certain age groups.

   a. The elderly (Ferrell 1991; Harkins et al. 1994; Parmelee et al. 1994):
      (1) Cognitive impairment complicating the history
      (2) Response biases
      (3) Multiple medications

   b. Children (McGrath and Unruh 1987; Ross and Ross 1988; Schechter et al. 1993; Houck et al. 1994; Chapter 28):
      (1) Verbal difficulties in the very young (including use of different scales)
      (2) Response to medications

B. Be able to perform an appropriate physical examination and to interpret physical findings that may be relevant to the pain complaint.

   1. Be familiar with the examination needed to define the organ system involved in a pain syndrome. The examination should involve, at a minimum, examining the site of pain, trying to reproduce the pain with physical maneuvers, and looking for obvious signs of dysfunction. Be able to refer to the appropriate specialist for further evaluation when any signs are discovered. Conversely, the assessor must be able to interpret the evaluations of specialists.
   2. Be aware of the underlying organic processes that may lead to pain (e.g., inflammation, nerve injury, tissue destruction).
   3. Be able to interpret physical findings that may be a result of treatment.
   4. Be aware of physical findings suggestive of secondary pain-perpetuating factors, such as sympathetically maintained and myofascial pain (Cailliet 1977; Travell and Simons 1983).

C. Know appropriate laboratory, electrophysiological, and radiographic procedures for pain evaluation.

   1. Understand that clinical evidence of a lesion does not necessarily mean that the lesion caused the pain; conversely, understand that absence of a lesion does not mean that the pain is psychogenic.
   2. Understand the scope and limitations of procedures for chronic pain patients sufficiently well to make a judicious selection of procedures and to prevent the discomfort and expense of unnecessary procedures.

D. Be able to use the patient's history, physical findings, and supporting tests to diagnose the underlying disease process and classify the pain complaint.

   1. Know the temporal classifications of pain (acute, recurrent, and chronic).
   2. Know the topographic classification of pain.

      a. Be able to distinguish among focal, radicular, referred, and central pain.
      b. Understand the patterns of pain distribution well enough to determine whether the pain is focal, referred, or central.

   3. Know the pathophysiological classifications of pain.

      a. Nociceptive pain is due to continuing tissue damage; nervous system is intact. Understand differences in presentation between somatic and visceral pain.
      b. Pain without active tissue damage may be due to neurological injury (neuropathic pain) or may be psychosocial in origin (psychogenic pain).

   4. Know syndromic classifications of pain. Understand the term *chronic nonmalignant pain syndrome*.

      a. Know the major cancer pain syndromes in adults and children (Chapter 23).
      b. Know common neuropathic pain syndromes in adults and children (Chapter 20).
      c. Know common nonmalignant medical illnesses in adults and children in which severe pain is a prominent and often undertreated feature (hemophilia, sickle-cell disease, acquired immunodeficiency syndrome).

II. An integrated approach to pain management

A. Know that optimal pain management requires a broad understanding of both nociceptive mechanisms and relevant psychosocial factors influencing treatment outcomes. Know the categories of potential pain-related interventions, their appropriate indications, and effective combinations of interventions.

B. Know the main pharmacologic approaches to pain management and the principles of pharmacodynamics and pharmacokinetics for infants, children, and adults (Chapters 7, 8, and 9).

C. Know the commonly used noninvasive neuroaugmentative techniques of pain management. Be aware of the data evaluating invasive measures of neuroaugmentation, including dorsal column stimulation and deep brain stimulation (Chapter 11).

D. Be familiar with local and regional anesthetic approaches to pain management (Chapter 13).

E. Know the commonly used surgical approaches to pain management. Be able to appropriately refer patients to specialists for evaluation and implementation of surgical procedures (Chapter 12).

F. Know physiatric approaches to pain management (Chapter 10).

   1. Know the analgesic potential of specific orthoses and prostheses and indications for their use.
   2. Understand the benefits of specific modalities of physical therapy, occupational therapy, and vocational training to chronic pain patients.

G. Know psychological techniques for pain management (Gatchell and Turk 1995; Chapter 15).

1. Know the spectrum of cognitive, behavioral, and other available psychotherapeutic interventions and be aware of specific indications that may warrant these approaches.
2. Be able to appropriately refer patients to specialists for evaluation and implementation of psychological approaches.

H. Know the multidisciplinary approach to the management of subacute and chronic pain and the data in support of its use (Rowlingson and Toomey 1988; Chapter 16).

I. Know that infants and children, like adults, require adequate pain control for acute treatment-related and postoperative pain. Know that potent opioids are appropriate for children and that painless routes of administration, if feasible, are advisable (Walco et al. 1994; Chapter 28).

J. Be aware of evidence that failure to treat pain in infants has adverse physiological consequences.

REFERENCES

American Psychiatric Association staff, Diagnostic and Statistical Manual of Mental Disorders: DSM-IV, American Psychiatric Association, Washington, D.C., 1994.

Bonica, J.J. (Ed.), The Management of Pain, 2nd ed., Lea & Febiger, Philadelphia, 1990.

Cailliet, R., Soft Tissue Pain and Disability, F.A. Davis Company, Philadelphia, 1977.

Ferrell, B.A., Pain management in elderly people, J. Am. Geriatr. Soc., 39(1) (1991) 64–73.

Fields, H.L., Evaluation of patients with persistent pain. In: H.L. Fields (Ed.), Pain, McGraw-Hill, New York, 1987, pp. 205–250.

France, R.D. and Krishnan, K.R.R., Pain in psychiatric disorders. In: R.D. France and K.R.R. Krishnan (Eds.), Chronic Pain, American Psychiatric Press, Washington, DC, 1988, pp. 116–141.

Gatchel, R.J. and Turk, D.C. (Eds.), Psychological Treatments for Pain: A Practitioner's Handbook, Guilford Press, New York, 1995.

Harkins, S.W., Price, D.D., Bush, F.M. and Small, R.E., Geriatric pain. In: P.D. Wall and R. Melzack (Eds.), Textbook of Pain, 3rd ed., Churchill Livingstone, Edinburgh, 1994, pp. 769–786.

Houck, C.S., Troshynski, T. and Berde, C.B., Treatment of pain in children. In: P.D. Wall and R. Melzack (Eds.), Textbook of Pain, 3rd ed., Churchill Livingstone, Edinburgh, 1994, pp. 1419–1436.

McGrath, P.A., Pain in Children: Nature, Assessment, and Treatment, Guilford Publications, New York, 1990.

McGrath, P.J. and Unruh, A., Pain in Children and Adolescents, Elsevier, Amsterdam, 1987.

Parmalee, P.A., Smith, B. and Katz, I.R., Pain complaints and cognitive status among elderly institution residents, J. Am. Geriatr. Soc., 41(5) (1993) 517–522.

Pilowsky, I., Pain and illness behavior assessment and management. In: P.D. Wall and R. Melzack (Eds.), Textbook of Pain, 3rd ed., Churchill Livingstone, Edinburgh, 1994, pp. 1309–1320.

Price, D.D., Psychological and Neural Mechanisms of Pain, Raven Press, New York, 1988.

Ross, D.M. and Ross, S.A., Childhood Pain: Current Issues, Research, and Management, Urban & Schwarzenberg, Baltimore, 1988.

Rowlingson, J.C. and Toomey, T.C., Multidisciplinary approaches to the management of cancer pain. In: J.N. Ghia (Ed.), The Multidisciplinary Pain Center, Kluwer Academic Publishers, Boston, 1988, pp. 45–73.

Schechter, N.L., Berde, C.B. and Yaster, M., Pain Management in Children and Adolescents, Williams & Wilkins, Baltimore, 1993.

Sternbach, R.A. (Ed.), The Psychology of Pain, 2nd ed., Raven Press, New York, 1986.

Travell, J.G. and Simons, D.G., Myofascial Pain and Dysfunction, The Trigger Point Manual, Williams & Wilkins, Baltimore, 1983.

Turk, D.C. and Melzack, R. (Eds.), Handbook of Pain Assessment, Guilford Press, New York, 1992.

Walco, G.A., Cassidy, R.C. and Schecter, N.L., Pain, hurt, and harm: the ethics of pain control in infants and children, N. Engl. J. Med., 331 (1994) 541–544.

Wall, P.D. and Melzack, R. (Eds.), Textbook of Pain, 3rd ed., Churchill Livingstone, Edinburgh, 1994.

Core Curriculum for Professional Education in Pain, edited by H.L. Fields, IASP Press, Seattle, © 1995.

6

Designing, Reporting, and Interpreting Clinical Trials of Treatments for Pain

I. Understand general principles of therapeutic studies.

  A. Understand the difference between two approaches in therapeutic trials: "explanatory" (an intent to derive a general biological principle, using highly selected subjects under optimal treatment conditions), and "pragmatic" (an intent to inform clinicians about the usefulness of the therapy under conditions approximating usual clinical practice) (Schwartz and Lellouch 1967).

  B. Be aware of the literature on the placebo effect, its variability, the factors that influence it, and the implications for clinical trials (Turner et al. 1994).

  C. Understand the relative advantages of prospectively collected vs. retrospectively collected data on treatment effectiveness (Friedman et al. 1985; Meinert 1986; Hulley and Cummings 1988).

  D. Understand various types of bias that can affect anecdotal observations by clinicians and understand the protection afforded by randomized assignment and blinding (Friedman et al. 1985; Meinert 1986; Hulley and Cummings 1988).

  E. Understand how drug side effects or other features of treatment may make perfect blinding impossible and introduce bias into studies. Be aware of measures that have been suggested to improve or validate blinding, including questionnaires regarding blinding, detailed assessment of side effects, and active placebos (Moscucci et al. 1987; Fisher and Greenberg 1993).

  F. Understand several reasons why order effects might be seen in therapeutic trials.

  G. Recognize the advantages and disadvantages of single-center and multicenter clinical trials (Friedman et al. 1985; Meinert 1986).

  H. Be familiar with the key clinical research design issues for studies of cognitive behavioral interventions for pain and pain behavior (e.g., progressive relaxation, imagery, activity scheduling, problem-solving techniques, operant techniques, changing maladaptive thoughts) (Holroyd and Creer 1986).

  I. Be familiar with steps to minimize bias in clinical trials of surgical techniques for pain control (North et al. 1993; North and Levy 1994).

  J. Be familiar with the terms "sensitivity" and "specificity" for a diagnostic test, particularly as they apply to tests that putatively predict response to chronic treatments (e.g., brief drug infusions to predict chronic treatment response).

II. Be familiar with specific choices made in the design of clinical trials of treatments for pain.

    A. Understand the relative advantages and disadvantages of various methods for measuring pain intensity and relief in clinical trials, including visual analog scales, verbal descriptor scales, and daily diaries, and how choices will vary with patient groups, length of study, and time course of treatment (Max and Laska 1991; Food and Drug Administration 1992; Turk and Melzack 1992).

    B. Recognize the problem posed by the fluctuation of pain levels in chronic pain conditions. Know the advantages and pitfalls of several possible solutions, such as averaging multiple assessments taken at different times and asking subjects to retrospectively average their pain over several preceding days or weeks (Jensen and McFarland 1993; Smith and Safer 1993).

    C. Be familiar with the multiple outcomes that need to be considered in "pragmatic" clinical trials, including pain intensity, pain duration, functional disability, medicine use, health care use and costs, psychological distress and well-being, and satisfaction with care (Spilker 1990; Turk and Melzack 1992).

    D. Understand the purpose of the usual treatment and control groups included in single-dose analgesic trials, including the test drug, placebo, and standard analgesic ("positive") control, and graded doses of test drug or standard. Be clear regarding the information provided by each of these comparisons, the risks of omitting them, and what is meant by the concept of "assay sensitivity" (Max and Laska 1991; Food and Drug Administration 1992).

    E. Understand the interpretation of analgesic trials in which rescue medication is routinely given (e.g., PCA studies or chronic cancer studies) (Portenoy 1991; Rosenblatt and Silverman 1992; Max 1994a).

    F. Be able to describe a "relative potency design," including its applicability to the comparative assessment of side effects at equianalgesic doses of two analgesics (Max and Laska 1991; Max 1994b).

    G. Understand the relative advantages and disadvantages of crossover vs. parallel group study designs, and understand the types of carryover effects that may occur in a crossover study (Bailar and Mosteller 1986; Max 1991).

    H. Be familiar with possible control conditions for evaluation of nondrug interventions for pain, including usual care, waiting list, information only, and sham-intervention control conditions (Holroyd and Creer 1986).

    I. Understand the types of study design used to assess dose-response relationships (Sheiner et al. 1989; Temple 1989).

    J. Understand the challenges for clinical trials posed by groups of patient whose pain is caused by several different mechanisms, and the design stratagems for addressing this problem (Max 1991).

III. Be familiar with basic statistical principles used in designing and evaluating clinical trials (Bailar and Mosteller 1986; Moore 1991).

    A. Understand the most common univariate tests used to assess the primary outcome, including the t-test, analysis of variance, tests to make comparisons among multiple experimental groups (e.g., Bonferroni's correction, Dunnett's test, Student-Newman-Keuls test), and the chi-square test.

B. Understand what is meant by statistical significance of a result, including p values and confidence intervals for an estimate of a variable.

C. Be familiar with how parametric and nonparametric tests differ and the occasions for using each.

D. Understand the statistical criticisms of the common two-period, two-treatment crossover design, and alternative crossover designs that may be better able to detect and estimate carryover effects (Bailar and Mosteller 1986; Jones and Kenward 1989; Max 1991; Ratkowsky et al. 1993).

E. Understand the method and limitations of power analyses to determine the sample size for a study.

F. Understand the bias that may be introduced if a study is stopped before the intended N is reached, and the reason that statistical penalties must be assessed for "multiple looks" (Friedman et al. 1985; Meinert 1986).

G. Understand the concept of "intent-to-treat" analysis and the types of bias that can result if data from treatment dropouts are excluded from the study report.

H. Understand the pitfalls of doing many statistical comparisons of many variables in a study, or of doing post-hoc analyses of study outcome in patient subsets.

I. Be familiar with the concepts of stratification and adaptive randomization in clinical trials, and their potential advantages (Friedman et al. 1985; Bailar and Mosteller 1986; Meinert 1986).

J. Be familiar with the concepts of single-case or "N of 1" designs (McQuay 1991) and "enriched enrollment" designs (Byas-Smith et al. 1995), including their potential advantages and pitfalls.

K. Be familiar with the advantages and pitfalls of meta-analyses (Jadad 1994).

L. Be familiar with the concept of treatment "effect size" in meta-analyses and how the effect size is calculated (Jadad 1994).

REFERENCES

Bailar, J.C. and Mosteller, F. (Eds.), Medical Uses of Statistics, NEJM Books, Waltham, MA, 1986.
Byas-Smith, M.G., Max, M.B., Muir, J. and Kingman, A., Transdermal clonidine compared to placebo in painful diabetic neuropathy using a two-stage "enriched enrollment" design, Pain, 60 (1995) 267–274.
Fisher, S. and Greenberg, R.P., How sound is the double-blind design for evaluating psychotropic drugs? J. Nerv. Ment. Dis., 181 (1993) 345–350.
Food and Drug Administration, Guideline for the Clinical Evaluation of Analgesic Drugs, U.S. Department of Health and Human Services, Rockville, MD, 1992.
Friedman L.M., Furberg, C.D. and DeMets, D.L., Fundamentals of Clinical Trials, 2nd ed., PSG Publishing, Littleton, MA, 1985.
Holroyd, K.A. and Creer, T.L., Self-management of Chronic Disease: Handbook of Clinical Interventions and Research, Academic Press, Orlando, 1986.
Hulley, S.B. and Cummings, S.R. (Eds.), Designing Clinical Research, Williams & Wilkins, Baltimore, 1988.

Jadad, A.R., Meta-analysis of randomised clinical trials in pain relief, D. Phil. Thesis, University of Oxford, 1994.
Jensen, M.P. and McFarland C.A., Increasing the reliability and validity of pain intensity measurement in chronic pain patients, Pain, 55 (1993) 195–204.
Jones, B. and Kenward, M.G., Design and Analysis of Cross-Over Trials, Chapman & Hall, New York, 1989.
Max, M.B., Neuropathic pain. In: M.B. Max, R.K. Portenoy and E.M. Laska (Eds.), The Design of Analgesic Clinical Trials, Progr. Pain Res. Ther, Vol. 18, Raven Press, New York, 1991, 193–219.
Max, M.B., Divergent traditions in analgesic clinical trials, Clin. Pharmacol. Ther., 56 (1994a) 237–241.
Max, M.B., Combining opioids with other drugs: challenges in clinical trial design. In: G.F. Gebhart, D.L. Hammond and T.S. Jensen (Eds.), Proceedings of the 7th World Congress on Pain, Progress in Pain Research and Management, Vol. 2, IASP Press, Seattle, 1994b, 569–586.

Max, M.B. and Laska, E.M., Single-dose comparisons. In: M.B. Max, R.K. Portenoy and E.M. Laska (Eds.), The Design of Analgesic Clinical Trials, Progress in Pain Research and Therapy, Vol. 18, Raven Press, New York, 1991, 55–96.

McQuay, H.J., N of 1 trials. In: M.B. Max, R.K. Portenoy and E.M. Laska (Eds.), The Design of Analgesic Clinical Trials, Progress in Pain Research and Therapy, Vol. 18, Raven Press, New York, 1991, 179–192.

Meinert, C.L., Clinical Trials: Design, Conduct, and Analysis, Oxford University Press, New York, 1986.

Moore, D.S., Statistics: Concepts and Controversies, 3rd ed., W.H. Freeman, New York, 1991.

Moscucci, M., Byrne, L., Weintraub, M. and Cox, C., Blinding, unblinding, and the placebo effect: an analysis of patients' guesses of treatment assignment in a double-blind trial, Clin. Pharmacol. Ther., 41 (1987) 259–265.

North, R.B. and Levy, R.M., Consensus conference on the neurosurgical management of pain, Neurosurgery, 34 (1994) 756–761.

North, R.B., Kidd, D.H., Zahurak, M., James, C.S. and Long, D., Spinal cord stimulation for chronic, intractable pain: experience over two decades, Neurosurgery, 32 (1993) 384–395.

Portenoy, R.K., Cancer pain. In: M.B. Max, R.K. Portenoy and E.M. Laska (Eds.), The Design of Analgesic Clinical Trials, Progress in Pain Research and Therapy, Vol. 18, Raven Press, New York, 1991, 233–265.

Ratkowsky, D.A., Evans, M.A. and Alldredge, J.R., Cross-Over Experiments: Design, Analysis, and Application, Marcel Dekker, New York, 1993.

Rosenblatt W.R. and Silverman, D.G., PCA as an investigative tool. In: R.S. Sinatra, L. Preble, A. Hord and B. Ginsberg (Eds.), Acute Pain: Mechanisms and Management, Mosby–Year Book, St. Louis, 1992, pp. 194–200.

Schwartz, D. and Lellouch, J., Explanatory and pragmatic attitudes in therapeutic trials, J. Chron. Dis., 20 (1967) 637–648.

Sheiner, L.B., Beal, S.L. and Sambol, N.C., Study designs for dose-ranging, Clin. Pharmacol. Ther., 46 (1989) 63–77.

Smith W.B. and Safer, M.A., The effect of present pain level on recall for pain and medication use, Pain, 55 (1993) 355–361.

Spilker, B. (Ed.), Quality of Life Assessment in Clinical Trials, Raven Press, New York, 1990.

Temple, R., Dose-response and registration of new drugs. In: L. Lasagna, S. Erill and C.A. Naranjo (Eds.), Dose-response Relationships in Clinical Pharmacology, Elsevier, Amsterdam, 1989, pp. 145–170.

Turk, D.C. and Melzack, R. (Eds.), Handbook of Pain Assessment, Guilford Press, New York, 1992.

Turner, J.A., Deyo, R.A., Loeser, J.D., Von Korff, M. and Fordyce, W.E., The importance of placebo effects in pain treatment and research, JAMA, 271 (1994) 1609–1614.

Core Curriculum for Professional Education in Pain, edited by H.L. Fields, IASP Press, Seattle, © 1995.

7

Drug Treatment I: Opioids

I. Understand the classification of opioid compounds (Jaffe and Martin 1990; Pasternak 1993).

A. Recognize those subclasses and specific drugs that are used clinically and are full agonists at the mu-opioid receptor:

1. Alkaloids (including semisynthetic alkaloids) such as morphine and codeine, hydromorphone, oxycodone, oxymorphone, codeine, heroin, hydrocodone, and dihydrocodeine
2. Synthetic opioids, including morphinan derivatives (such as levorphanol), phenylpiperidine derivatives (such as fentanyl, sufentanil, alfentanil, and meperidine), and diphenylheptane derivatives (such as methadone and propoxyphene)

B. Recognize those opioid drugs that are used clinically and are partial agonists at the mu receptor:

1. Semisynthetic alkaloids, including buprenorphine
2. Synthetic opioids, including the morphinan dezocine
3. Tramadol (which also has nonopioid analgesic effects)

C. Recognize those opioid drugs that are used clinically and are known as the mixed agonists-antagonists because they possess antagonist activity at the mu-opioid receptor and agonist activity at another opioid receptor subtype (e.g., kappa receptor):

1. Semisynthetic alkaloids, including nalbuphine
2. Synthetic opioids, including benzomorphan derivatives (such as pentazocine) and morphinan derivatives (such as butorphanol)

D. Recognize those opioid drugs that are used clinically and are pure antagonists of the opioid receptor, including:

1. Naloxone
2. Naltrexone

E. Recognize the major classes of the endorphins, or endogenous opioid compounds, and know the precursor molecules for each.

1. The precursor proopiomelanocortin yields beta endorphin.
2. The precursor prodynorphin yields the dynorphin peptides.
3. The precursor proenkephalin yields the enkephalin peptides.

II. Know those aspects of basic opioid pharmacology that are relevant to the use of opioid drugs in clinical practice.

A. Be aware of the common structure shared by all opioids and how modifications of this structure alter the activities of the resulting compounds (Jaffe and Martin 1990; Carr et al. 1991; Pasternak 1993).

B. Be aware of the importance of physical properties of opioid drugs (Jaffe and Martin 1990).

    1. Understand how the lipid solubility of an opioid influences its pharmacokinetics.

    2. Understand the particular importance of lipid solubility in determining the pharmacodynamics following intraspinal administration (Cousins et al. 1988).

C. Be aware of major findings related to opioid receptor pharmacology (Jaffe and Martin 1990; Pasternak 1993; Reisine and Bell 1993; Dickenson 1994).

    1. The major types of opioid receptors (mu, kappa, and delta), their subtypes, and the receptor-selective actions that have been identified
    2. Localization of opioid receptors in relation to sites likely to be involved in analgesia
    3. Cloning and molecular characterization of opioid receptors as members of the G protein receptor superfamily (Reisine and Bell 1993)
    4. The localization of opioid receptors outside the nervous system and the implications of this localization for widespread involvement of opioid mechanisms in the physiologic functioning of many organ systems, including cardiovascular, gastrointestinal, and immune system (Jaffe and Martin 1990; Dickenson 1994; Stein 1994)
    5. The intracellular events produced by binding of the opioid receptor, including activation of second-messenger systems (e.g., G protein, protein kinase C), interaction with other receptors (e.g., N-methyl-D-aspartate), and electrophysiologic outcomes (e.g., hyperpolarization due to opening of potassium channels or closing of calcium channels) (Pasternak 1993; Dickenson 1994; Mayer et al. 1995)

D. Understand tolerance and physical dependence (Cox 1991; Yaksh 1991; Mayer et al. 1995; Portenoy 1994b).

    1. Be able to define tolerance and physical dependence.
    2. Recognize the multiple types of tolerance (e.g., associative or behavioral vs. nonassociative or pharmacologic) and that tolerance can develop to any opioid effect.
    3. Be aware of the multiple mechanisms that may be responsible for opioid tolerance or physical dependence.
    4. Be able to define intrinsic efficacy and understand that this property may be involved in the development of tolerance and the variable degree of cross-tolerance observed when one opioid is changed to another.

E. Recognize that the mechanisms that produce tolerance are not the only factors that can reduce opioid efficacy and that the following pathological processes, which have the same result, may be more important clinically (Dickenson 1994; Portenoy 1994b):

    1. Increased nociception due to progression of a tissue-damaging lesion
    2. Sensitization of central nervous system neurons, rendering them less responsive to opioid mechanisms
    3. Transmission of nociceptive information along afferent pathways that are usually non-nociceptive and are less subject to modulation by opioid mechanisms

4. Pharmacokinetic processes, such as the production of active metabolites that may have anti-analgesic effects

F. Recognize that individual variation in metabolic processes may be genetically determined and influence the efficacy or toxicity of opioid drugs.

1. Variability in the activity of the P450 enzyme, 2D6, influences the endogenous conversion of codeine to morphine and oxycodone to oxymorphone.
2. Variability in the glucuronidation of morphine influences the ratio of active glucuronidated metabolites to parent compound.

III. Know those aspects of clinical opioid pharmacology that are relevant to the use of opioid drugs in patient care (Benedetti 1990; Jaffe and Martin 1990; Portenoy et al. 1990; American Pain Society 1992; Carr et al. 1992; Foley 1993; Jacox et al. 1994).

A. Be able to define the terms efficacy, maximal efficacy, relative efficacy, responsiveness, potency, and relative potency (Portenoy 1994b).

B. Understand the differences in clinical effects among pure opioid agonists, partial agonists, mixed agonists-antagonists, and antagonists.

1. Be aware that the existence of a ceiling effect for analgesia and the lack of oral formulations limit the utility of the partial agonist and mixed agonist-antagonist drugs for the management of chronic pain.
2. Be aware that the mixed agonist-antagonist opioids are more likely to cause psychotomimetic effects than are the pure agonist opioids.
3. Be aware that the partial agonists and mixed agonist-antagonist drugs have a ceiling effect for respiratory depression, in contrast to the pure agonist opioids.
4. Be aware that abstinence can be precipitated when a partial agonist or mixed agonist-antagonist is administered to a patient who is physically dependent on a pure agonist drug.

C. Recognize the great individual variability in opioid pharmacokinetics and pharmacodynamics and understand that this variability, combined with changes in responsiveness over time, mandates individualization of opioid doses based on a continuing process of assessment (analgesia and side effects) and dose titration (American Pain Society 1992; Carr et al. 1992; Foley 1993; Jacox et al. 1994).

D. Be aware of the varied routes of administration by which opioids can be delivered:

1. Oral
2. Sublingual
3. Rectal
4. Transdermal
5. Subcutaneous via intermittent injection or continuous infusion
6. Intramuscular via intermittent injection
7. Intravenous via intermittent injection or continuous infusion
8. Spinal epidural via intermittent injection or continuous infusion
9. Spinal subarachnoid via intermittent injection or continuous infusion
10. Intraventricular

E. Understand the clinical factors that influence the decision to use specific routes of administration in the management of acute and chronic pain (Carr et al. 1992; Jacox et al. 1994).

   1. Be aware of the efficacy and utility of noninvasive routes, particularly the oral route, when treating chronic pain.
   2. Be aware that the need for rapid onset of analgesia may justify the parenteral route.
   3. Be aware that infusions can eliminate bolus effects (peak concentration toxicity or pain recurrence at the end of the dosing interval).
   4. Be aware that patient-controlled analgesia can provide appropriate patients an effective means to continually adjust treatment to meet analgesic needs.
   5. Be aware that intraspinal administration (epidural or subarachnoid) may be able to reduce the opioid side effects associated with systemic opioid administration.

F. Be aware of the equianalgesic dose tables derived from relative potency data and recognize the need to adjust doses when changing drugs or routes of administration (American Pain Society 1992; Carr et al. 1992; Jacox et al. 1994).

G. Understand major pharmacokinetic and pharmacodynamic considerations for each opioid drug and for each formulation and route of administration used clinically.

   1. Know important pharmacokinetic information for each drug (Jaffe and Martin 1990).

      a. Elimination half-life
      b. Existence of active metabolites, particularly for meperidine (with its toxic metabolite, normeperidine) and morphine (with its active opioid metabolite, morphine-6-glucuronide)
      c. Influence of patient characteristics, including age (changes associated with very young age and old age) and major organ dysfunction (changes associated with disease of the kidneys or liver)

   2. Know relevant pharmacokinetic and pharmacodynamic information for each formulation and route of administration (Benedetti 1990; Portenoy et al. 1990; American Pain Society 1992; Carr et al. 1992; Foley 1993; Jacox et al. 1994).

      a. Bioavailability
      b. Time-action profile for a single dose, including time of onset, time to peak effect, and duration of effect
      c. Time-action profile for repeated doses and infusions, including time of onset and time to approach steady state

H. Be aware of the potential for additive analgesic effects that can occur with the combination of opioids and other drugs.

   1. Systemic opioids combined with nonopioid analgesics or adjuvant analgesics
   2. Intraspinal opioids combined with local anesthetics

I. Recognize that specific clinical guidelines have been recommended for different patient populations and that the techniques needed for optimal therapy differ for the following conditions:

   1. Postoperative and procedure-related acute pain (Benedetti 1990; American Pain Society 1992; Carr et al. 1992)
   2. Cancer-related pain (American Pain Society 1992; Jacox et al. 1994)

3. Chronic nonmalignant pain (Schug et al. 1991; Portenoy 1994a)
4. Chronic or recurrent pain due to medical illness (e.g., arthritis, sickle cell anemia, headache, HIV/AIDS)

J. Be aware of the potential side effects and toxicities of opioid drugs (Cousins et al. 1988; Jaffe and Martin 1990; American Pain Society 1992; Carr et al. 1992; Jacox et al. 1994).

1. Know the clinical presentation and management strategies for common side effects, including constipation, nausea, somnolence, mental clouding, and urinary retention.
2. Know that respiratory depression is rare during chronic opioid use.
3. Be aware that side effects and toxicity may be more likely with specific patient characteristics such as advanced age, major organ dysfunction (e.g., renal disease, chronic encephalopathy, chronic obstructive pulmonary disease), and concurrent centrally acting drugs (e.g., benzodiazepines).

K. Understand the use of naloxone to treat acute opioid overdose.

1. Know the risks associated with naloxone administration to patients receiving chronic opioid therapy, including abstinence and recurrent pain, and understand the value of careful titration using a dilute solution of naloxone (Jacox et al. 1994).
2. Be aware that naloxone should only be given to patients receiving chronic opioid therapy to reverse respiratory depression or impending respiratory depression.
3. Know that naloxone has a short half-life and that repeated injections or an infusion are usually needed to treat opioid overdose.

L. Understand that the risk of abstinence mandates dose tapering after a few days of frequent dosing with an opioid drug, and be aware of the techniques used to discontinue these drugs safely, including the rate of the taper, substitution-withdrawal with a long half-life opioid, and the use of clonidine to prevent abstinence.

M. Know the definition of addiction (i.e., loss of control over drug use, compulsive use, and continued use despite harm) and understand the implications of the therapeutic use of a potential drug of abuse (Portenoy 1994).

1. Understand the need to monitor the patient for the appearance of aberrant drug-related behavior during chronic therapy.
2. Be aware of the various diagnoses that may account for aberrant drug-related behavior and understand the assessment that is needed to accurately characterize the patient's response.
3. Be aware of the approaches to the management of the patient who exhibits aberrant, drug-related behavior during long-term opioid treatment of chronic pain.

REFERENCES

American Pain Society, Principles of Analgesic Use in the Treatment of Acute and Chronic Cancer Pain, 3rd ed., American Pain Society, Skokie, IL, 1992.

Benedetti, C., Acute pain: a review of its effects and therapy with systemic opioids. In: C. Benedetti, C.R. Chapman and G. Giron (Eds.), Opioid Analgesia: Recent Advances in Systemic Administration, Advances in Pain Research and Therapy, Vol. 14, Raven, New York, 1990, pp. 367–424.

Carr, D.B., Jacox, A.K., Chapman, C.R., et al., Acute Pain Management: Operative or Medical Procedures and Trauma, Clinical Practice Guideline, AHCPR Pub. No. 92-0032, U.S. Department of Health and Human Services, Public Health Service, Agency for Health Care Policy and Research, Rockville, MD, 1992.

Carr, D.B., Lipkowski, A.W. and Silbert, B.S., Biochemistry of the opioid peptides. In: F.G. Estafanous (Ed.), Opioids in Anesthesia II, Butterworth-Heinemann, Boston, 1991.

Cousins, M.J., Cherry, D.A. and Gourlay, G.K., Acute and chronic pain: use of spinal opioids. In: M.J. Cousins and P.O. Bridenbaugh (Eds.), Neural Blockade in Clincal Anesthesia and Pain Management, 2nd ed., Lippincott, Philadlephia, 1988, pp. 955–1029.

Cox, B.M., Molecular and cellular mechanisms in opioid tolerance. In: A.I. Basbaum and J.-M. Besson (Eds.), Towards a New Pharmacotherapy of Pain, John Wiley & Sons, New York, 1991, pp. 137–156.

Dickenson, A.H., Where and how do opioids act? In: G.F. Gebhart, D.L. Hammond and T.S. Jensen (Eds.), Proceedings of the 7th World Congress on Pain, Progress in Pain Research and Management, Vol. 2, IASP Press, Seattle, 1994, pp. 525–552.

Foley, K.M., Opioid analgesics in clinical pain management. In: A. Herz (Ed.), Handbook of Experimental Pharmacology, Vol. 104/II, Springer-Verlag, Berlin, 1993, pp. 697–742.

Jacox, A.K., Carr, D.B., Payne, R., et al., Management of Cancer Pain, Clinical Practice Guideline No. 9, AHCPR Pub. No. 94-0592, U.S. Department of Health and Human Services, Public Health Service, Agency for Health Care Policy and Research, Rockville, MD, 1994.

Jaffe, J.H. and Martin, W.R., Opioid analgesics and antagonists. In: A.G. Gilman, T.W. Rall, A.S. Niesf and P. Taylor (Eds.), The Pharmacological Basis of Therapeutics, 8th ed., Pergamon Press, New York, 1990, pp. 485–521.

Mayer, D.J., Mao, J. and Price, D.D., The development of morphine tolerance and dependence is associated with translocation of protein kinase C, Pain, 61 (1995) 365–374.

Pasternak, G.W., Pharmacological mechanisms of opioid analgesics, Clin. Neuropharmacol., 16 (1993) 1–18.

Portenoy, R.K., Opioid therapy for chronic nonmalignant pain: current status. In: H.L. Fields and J.C. Liebeskind (Eds.), Pharmacological Approaches to the Treatment of Chronic Pain: New Concepts and Critical Issues, Progress in Pain Research and Management, Vol. 1, IASP Press, Seattle, 1994a, pp. 247–288.

Portenoy, R.K., Opioid tolerance and responsiveness: research findings and clincal observations. In: G.F. Gebhart, D.L. Hammond and T.S. Jensen (Eds.), Proceedings of the 7th World Congress on Pain, Progress in Pain Research and Management, Vol. 2, IASP Press, Seattle, 1994b, pp. 595–619.

Portenoy, R.K., Foley, K.M. and Inturrisi, C.E., The nature of opioid responsiveness and its implications for chronic pain: new hypotheses derived from studies of opioid infusions, Pain, 43 (1990) 273–286.

Reisine, T. and Bell, G.I., Molecular biology of opioid receptors, Trends Neurosci., 16 (1993) 506–510.

Schug, S.A, Merry, A.F. and Acland, R.H., Treatment principles for the use of opioids in pain of nonmalignant origin, Drugs, 42 (1991) 228–239.

Stein, C., Interaction of immune-competent cells and nociceptors. In: G.F. Gebhart, D.L. Hammond and T.S. Jensen (Eds.), Proceedings of the 7th World Congress on Pain, Progress in Pain Research and Management, Vol. 2, IASP Press, Seattle, 1994, pp. 285–297.

Yaksh, T.L, Tolerance: factors involved in changes in the dose-effect relationship with chronic drug exposure. In: A.I. Basbaum and J.-M. Besson (Eds.), Towards a New Pharmacotherapy of Pain, John Wiley & Sons, New York, 1991, pp. 157–180.

Core Curriculum for Professional Education in Pain, edited by H.L. Fields, IASP Press, Seattle, © 1995.

8

Drug Treatment II: Antipyretic Analgesics, i.e., Non-steroidals, Acetaminophen, and Phenazone Derivatives

I. Pharmacodynamics (Paulus 1985; Taiwo and Levine 1988; Kantor 1989; Handwerker 1991; McCormack and Brune 1991; Brune et al. 1992; Malmberg and Yaksh 1992; Williams 1993; Dray 1994; Laneuville et al. 1994; McCormack 1994; Neugebauer et al. 1994; Vane et al. 1994).

   A. Know the following about nonsteroidal anti-inflammatory drugs (NSAIDs):

   1. All NSAIDs or their active metabolites are acids. These acids accumulate in inflamed tissue, the gastrointestinal tract (GI) tract, the kidney, and the bone marrow.
   2. NSAIDs inhibit cyclooxygenase (COX1 and COX2), which produce prostaglandins from arachidonic acid.
   3. Prostaglandins sensitize nociceptors to the actions of other mediators of pain (histamine, bradykinin, H^+ ions) in the periphery and facilitate pain-related neuronal activities in the spinal cord.
   4. NSAIDs reduce leukocyte invasion in inflamed tissue.
   5. NSAIDs enhance the production of leukotrienes from arachidonic acid.
   6. Leukotrienes are mediators of pseudoallergic and allergic reactions.

   B. Know the characteristics of nonacidic antipyretic analgesics, i.e., acetaminophen, phenazone, propyphenazone, and dipyrone (active metabolites of 4-methylaminophenazone and others):

   1. Are weak bases or neutral substances
   2. Penetrate easily into the central nervous system (CNS) and reach equally high concentrations throughout the body
   3. Are weak inhibitors of cyclooxygenases
   4. Enhance leukotriene production
   5. Exert their main actions in the CNS (inhibition of pain and fever); the mediators involved are not fully defined.
   6. Dipyrone has some antispasmodic action.

II. Pharmacokinetics

   A. Be aware of the following properties of NSAIDs:

   1. With some, absorption begins in the stomach (aspirin, hydrolyzed, and unhydrolyzed); all others are absorbed in the small intestine.
   2. For some, parenteral administration is possible.
   3. Speed of onset of action is dependent on the speed of absorption.

4. Mostly unchanged at elimination, ususally after conjugation reactions (salicylic acid, diflunisal, ketoprofen, indomethacin) or by conjugation after oxidation (diclofenac, ibuprofen, piroxicam, and most others)
5. Show different elimination half-lives: short half-life (one to six hours) for diclofenac, flurbiprofen, ibuprofen, and ketoprofen; intermediate half-life (about 12 to 24 hours) for naproxen, diflunisal, and nabumetone (active metabolite); long half-life (days) for piroxicam, phenylbutazone, and tenoxicam
6. Their elimination is retarded in the elderly.
7. Interactions with other acids in plasma protein binding and tubular excretion

B. Be aware of the following properties of acetaminophen and phenazone derivatives:

1. They are absorbed in the small intestine (acetaminophen, dipyrone).
2. Parenteral administration is possible.
3. They are metabolized in the liver; half-life is two hours for acetaminophen, five to 25 hours for phenazone, and two to 10 hours for propyphenazone and dipyrone.
4. Elimination occurs by renal excretion of the metabolites.
5. Elimination is retarded in liver disease and in the elderly.

III. Know the side effects and drug interactions for (Brune and Lanz 1985; Paulus 1985; Murray and Brater 1993; Figueras et al. 1994; Langman et al. 1994):

A. NSAIDs

1. GI tract: irritations (10%), bleeding ulcerations, perforations (1 per 10,000); serious side effects are least prominent with ibuprofen, most prominent with azapropazone and piroxicam
2. Kidney damage: occasional
3. Liver damage: occasional, particularly seen with aspirin (in children) and diclofenac (in adults)
4. Bone marrow damage: aplastic anemia (most prominent with phenylbutazone)
5. Pseudoallergic reactions (10%, particularly in asthmatics, patients with neurodermitis, and children with nasal polyposis and related conditions)
6. Hypotension
7. Occasional severe allergic reactions (Steven's Johnson syndrome, Lyell syndrome, shock)
8. Aspirin: inhibition of platelet aggregation for days, cofactor in Reye's syndrome in children
9. Ketorolac: inhibition (for days) of platelet aggregation

B. Acetaminophen, phenazone, and derivatives

1. Acetaminophen

   a. Liver damage with overdosage
   b. Long-term effects in patients abusing combinations (analgesic nephropathy, urinary tract tumors)

2. Phenazone and derivatives

   a. Allergic skin reactions (frequent) and pseudoallergic reactions (rare severe skin reactions)
   b. Risk of agranulocytosis low but real (1 per 100,000 weekly treatment periods for dipyrone)
   c. Shock cases occasional, as with NSAIDs

IV. Know the major indications for use (Kantor 1989; McCormack and Brune 1991; Brune et al. 1992; Levy et al. 1995):

A. NSAIDs

1. Chronic intensive inflammatory pain, e.g., rheumatoid arthritis (diclofenac, indomethacin, piroxicam)
2. Phasic intensive inflammatory pain as in osteoarthrosis (diclofenac, ibuprofen, ketoprofen; short half-life)
3. Acute posttraumatic or postoperative pain (diclofenac, flurbiprofen, ibuprofen, ketoprofen; short half-life)
4. Headache (ibuprofen, ketoprofen, naproxen)
5. Dysmenorrhea

B. Acetaminophen

1. Some forms of headache
2. Fever (e.g., in children)

REFERENCES

Brune, K. and Lanz, R., Pharmacokinetics of nonsteroidal anti-inflammatory drugs. In: I.L. Bonta, M.A. Bray and M.J. Parnham (Eds.), Handbook of Inflammation, Elsevier Science Publishers B.V., Amsterdam, 1985, pp. 413–449.

Brune, K., Geisslinger, G. and Menzel-Soglowek, S., Pure enantiomers of 2-arylpropionic acids: tools in pain research and improved drugs in rheumatology, J. Clin. Pharmacol., 32 (1992) 944–952.

Dray, A., Tasting the inflammatory soup: the role of peripheral neurons, Pain Review, 1 (1994) 153–171.

Figueras, A., Capell, D., Castel, J.M. and Laporte, J.R., Spontaneous reporting of adverse drug reactions to nonsteroidal anti-inflammatory drugs, Eur. J. Clin. Pharmacol., 47 (1994) 297–303.

Handwerker, H.O., What peripheral mechanisms contribute to nociceptive transmission and hyperalgesia? In: A.L. Basbaum and J.L. Besson (Eds.), Towards a New Pharmacotherapy of Pain, John Wiley & Sons, Chichester, 1991, pp. 5–19.

Kantor, T.G., Concepts in pain control, Semin. Arthritis Rheum., 18 (1989) 94–99.

Laneuville, O., Breuer, D.K., Dewitt, D.L., Hla, T., Funk, C.D. and Smith, W.L., Differential inhibition of human prostaglandin endoperoxide H synthases-1 and -2 by nonsteroidal anti-inflammatory drugs, J. Pharmacol. Exp. Ther., 271 (1994) 927–934.

Langman, M.J.S., Weil, J., Wainwright, P., Lawson, D.H., Rawlings, M.D., Logan, R.F.A., Murphy, M., Vessey, M.P. and Colin-Jones, D.G., Risks of bleeding peptic ulcer associated with individual nonsteroidal anti-inflammatory drugs, Lancet, 343 (1994) 1075–1078.

Levy, M., Zylber-Katz, E. and Rosenkranz, B., Clinical pharmacokinetics of dipyrone and its metabolites, Clin. Pharmacokinet., 28 (1995) 216–234.

Malmberg, A.B. and Yaksh, T.L., Antinociceptive actions of spinal nonsteroidal anti-inflammatory agents on the formalin test in the rat, Journal of Experimental Therapeutics, 263 (1992) 136–146.

McCormack, K., Nonsteroidal anti-inflammatory drugs and spinal nociceptive processing, Pain, 59 (1994) 9–44.

McCormack, K. and Brune K., Dissociation between antinociceptive and inflammatory effects of the nonsteroidal anti-inflammatory drugs, Drugs, 41 (1991) 533–545.

Murray, M.D. and Brater, D.C., Renal toxicity of the nonsteroidal anti-inflammatory drugs, Annu. Rev. Pharmacol. Toxicol., 32 (1993) 435–465.

Neugebauer, V., Schaible, H.-G., He, X., Lücke, T., Gündling, P. and Schmidt, R.F., Electrophysiological evidence for a spinal antinociceptive action of dipyrone, Agents Actions, 41 (1994) 62–70.

Paulus, H.E., FDA arthritis advisory committee meeting: postmarketing surveillance of nonsteroidal antiinflammatory drugs, Arthritis Rheum., 28 (1985) 1168–1169.

Shimada, S.G., Otterness, I.G. and Stitt, J.T., A study of the mechanism of action of the mild analgesic dipyrone, Agents Actions, 41 (1994) 188–192.

Taiwo, Y.O. and Levine, J.D., Prostaglandins inhibit endogenous pain control mechanisms by blocking transmission at spinal noradrenergic synapses, J. Neurosci., 8 (1988) 1346–1349.

Vane, J.R., Mitchell, J.A., Appleton, I., Tomlinson, A., Bishop-Bailey, D., Croxtall, J. and Willoughby, D.A., Inducible isoforms of cyclooxygenase and nitric-oxide synthase in inflammation, Proc. Natl. Acad. Sci. USA, 91 (1994) 2046–2050.

Verbeeck, R.K., Pharmacokinetic drug interactions with nonsteroidal anti-inflammatory drugs, Clin. Pharmacokinet., 19 (1990) 44–66.

Williams, K.M., Breit, S. and Day, R.O., Biochemical actions and clinical pharmacology of anti-inflammatory drugs, Advances in Drug Research, 24 (1993) 121–152.

Core Curriculum for Professional Education in Pain, edited by H.L. Fields, IASP Press, Seattle, © 1995.

9

Drug Treatment III: Antidepressants, Anticonvulsants, and Miscellaneous Agents

I. Antidepressants (Couch et al. 1976; Watson 1982; Stambaugh and Lance 1983; Blackwell 1987; Ray et al. 1987; Max et al. 1988; Portenoy 1990; Sindrup et al. 1990b; Magni 1991; Max et al. 1992; Onghena and Van Houdenhove 1992; Sindrup et al. 1992; Carette et al. 1994; Glassman and Roose 1994; Max 1994)

A. Know the indications for the use of antidepressants.

1. Be aware of those syndromes for which support for the use of these drugs derives from controlled studies (e.g., migraine and tension headaches, postherpetic neuralgia, diabetic neuropathy, fibromyalgia, poststroke pain).
2. Be aware of indications supported by anecdotal experience (cancer pain with continuous neuropathic component).
3. Be aware that a clinical diagnosis of depression is not a requirement for use of antidepressants for pain.

B. Know the specific drugs used for the treatment of pain.

1. Know which drugs have analgesic efficacy proven by controlled trials (amitriptyline, desipramine, nortriptyline, imipramine, doxepin).
2. Know drugs for which supporting data is only anecdotal.
3. Be aware of the major hypotheses to explain the efficacy of the tricyclic antidepressants, and of the mixed results in studies of serotonin-specific reuptake inhibitors in neuropathic pain.
4. Know the major pharmacological differences between the commonly used antidepressant medications.

C. Be aware of principles of dosing antidepressants in the treatment of pain.

1. Know the usual dosage range and know the difference between this and antidepressant doses.
2. Understand the importance and have practical knowledge of dose titration.
3. When available, understand the value of blood levels in assessing optimum dose, potential toxicity, and compliance with therapy. Know that blood levels vary greatly in patients taking identical doses. Know that blood levels vary greatly in patients taking identical doses.
4. Be able to choose an appropriate endpoint for dosing, recognizing its empiric nature, e.g., intolerable side effects or blood level in the toxic range.
5. Understand the potential value in switching from one drug to another in the case of therapeutic failure.
6. Know demographic, metabolic, or disease-related factors that may affect on drug selection or dose titration (e.g., age, renal or hepatic disease, preexistent chronic or acute encephalopathy, or use of drugs with sedative or anticholinergic effects).

D. Know the common side effects of the antidepressant drugs used in the treatment of pain (e.g., sedation, dry mouth, memory impairment, urinary retention, orthostatic hypotension, and cardiac conduction abnormalities with tricyclic antidepressants).

E. Be aware of the possibility that the quinidine-like effects of tricyclic antidepressants might increase the risk of malignant arrhythmias in patients with coronary ischemia.

II. Anticonvulsant drugs (Swerdlow 1984; Killian and Fromm 1988; Portenoy 1990)

A. Know the indications for the use of anticonvulsant drugs.

1. Know those syndromes for which the use of these drugs is supported in controlled studies (e.g., trigeminal neuralgia, diabetic neuropathy, the lancinating pain of postherpetic neuralgia).
2. Know those syndromes for which these drugs are suggested in anecdotal series (other neuropathic pains with a lancinating component, poststroke pain).

B. Know that, in addition to carbamazepine, drugs such as phenytoin, valproate, clonazepam, gabapentin, and other new anticonvulsants may be useful.

C. Know the appropriate dosing regimen for each anticonvulsant used as an adjuvant analgesic.

1. Understand the similarity between dosing for analgesic purposes and anticonvulsant dosing.
2. For phenytoin, understand the value of an oral loading dose and how to implement it.
3. For carbamazepine, valproate, and clonazepam, understand the importance of low initial doses and gradual upward titration to avoid intolerable side effects.
4. Understand the value of blood levels in monitoring patient compliance, levels associated with effective analgesia, and potential explanations for failure.

D. Know potential toxicities of these drugs and possible monitoring schemes for detecting toxicity (e.g., aplastic anemia from carbamazepine and felbamate).

III. Neuroleptics (Beaver et al. 1966; Ray et al. 1987)

A. Know indications for neuroleptics when used as adjuvant analgesics.

1. Know that methotrimeprazine is the only neuroleptic with analgesic potential supported by controlled studies.
2. Know the anecdotal evidence for their use in neuropathic pain.
3. Understand their potential value in treating patients with coexistent symptoms, such as nausea or anxiety.
4. Be aware of the lack of a theoretical basis for analgesic effects of neuroleptics, and that the evidence for their efficacy is controversial at best.

B. Know the dosing regimens used for neuroleptics in the treatment of pain.

C. Be aware of the potential toxicities of the neuroleptic drugs.

1. Know the potential for long-term, refractory movement disorders (the tardive syndromes) and consider this risk in the long-term administration of these drugs.

    2. Be aware of the short-term, reversible toxicity, including other movement disorders (e.g., dystonic reactions), sedation, orthostatic hypotension, etc.

    3. Be aware that combining neuroleptics with tricyclic antidepressants may produce additive toxicity because of overlapping side effects.

IV. Antihistamines (Stambaugh and Lance 1983; Rumore and Schlichting 1986)

    A. Be aware of the literature supporting the use of antihistamines, specifically hydroxyzine, orphenadrine, and diphenhydramine, as analgesics.

    B. Recognize the limited role played by these drugs in clinical pain management and know some of the potential reasons (questionable long-term efficacy, questionable analgesia at the lower doses clinically tolerated).

    C. Understand the potential utility of hydroxyzine in cancer pain when used to treat concurrent symptoms of nausea or anxiety.

V. Analeptic drugs (Forrest et al. 1977; Bruera et al. 1987)

    A. Be aware of the literature supporting the analgesic potential of analeptic drugs (controlled trials of dextroamphetamine in experimental pain and postoperative pain, controlled trial of methylphenidate in cancer pain).

    B. Understand the reasons for the limited role played by these drugs in the management of nonmalignant pain (e.g., possible tachyphylaxis on long-term administration, potential for change in personality, insomnia, and cardiac toxicity).

    C. Understand the potential value of these drugs in the treatment of cancer pain with coexistent opioid-induced sedation.

VI. Corticosteroids (Kozin et al. 1981; Devor et al. 1985; Bruera et al. 1987)

    A. Understand the literature supporting the use of corticosteroids as analgesics.

        1. Know the role of these drugs in the management of cancer pain and other symptoms (controlled studies in pain and nausea, anecdotal reports in lassitude, anorexia, and others).

        2. Be aware of the anecdotal reports supporting the use of corticosteroids in reflex sympathetic dystrophy.

        3. Be aware of the laboratory evidence supporting the use of steroids in stabilizing function of injured nerves.

    B. Understand the reasons for the limited role played by these drugs in most nonmalignant pain syndromes and their substantial potential for toxicity with short-term or long-term use.

VII. Muscle relaxants (Bercel 1977; Ray et al. 1987; Max et al. 1988; Portenoy 1990; Carette et al. 1994; Dellemijn and Fields 1994)

    A. Know the potential indications for muscle relaxants as a short-term treatment for muscle spasm from a variety of causes.

    B. Know the specific drugs used as muscle relaxants.

        1. Be aware of "true" muscle relaxants used for spasticity (e.g., dantrolene, diazepam, baclofen).
        2. Be aware of drugs used for muscle spasm that are not true antispasticity agents (e.g., carisoprodol, methocarbomol, cyclobenzaprine)

    C. Know the data supporting the use of muscle relaxant drugs for common musculoskeletal pain problems.

        1. Be aware of the paucity of controlled studies.
        2. Be aware of the evidence for short-term salutary effects but the lack of evidence for long-term administration.
        3. Understand that drug selection is empirical.

    D. Know the appropriate dosing regimens and toxicity associated with these drugs.

VIII. Sympatholytic drugs (Abram and Lightfoot 1981; Ghostine et al. 1984; Arner 1991; Raja 1991; Dellemijn et al. 1994)

    A. Know the rationale for the use of sympatholytic drugs in the management of sympathetically maintained pain.

    B. Know the data that supports the use of sympatholytic drugs by a variety of routes for management of sympathetically maintained pain.

        1. Be aware of the anecdotal and single-blind controlled evidence that intravenous phentolamine may be useful as an aid in diagnosis of sympathetically maintained pain and its treatment.
        2. Be aware of the limited anecdotal evidence for oral phenoxybenzamine, prazosin, terazosin, and other oral sympatholytic agents.
        3. Be aware of the anecdotal and limited controlled evidence for regional intravenous administration of guanethidine or bretylium.

    C. Understand the potential confounding factors and controversies surrounding interpretation of pain relief from each route of administration.

    D. Know the dosing regimens and toxicities of these medications.

IX. Local anesthetics and antiarrhythmics (IMPACT 1984; Lindstrom and Lindblom 1987; Dejgard et al. 1988; Chabal et al. 1989; Portenoy 1990; Rowbotham et al. 1991; Chabal et al. 1992; Stracke et al. 1992; Galer et al. 1993)

    A. Be aware of the evidence demonstrating the efficacy of oral tocainide and mexiletine in neuropathic pain.

B. Know the rationale for the use of these drugs in neuropathic pain.

   1. Understand that they block voltage-dependent sodium channels, as do certain anticonvulsants (e.g., carbamazepine and valproate).
   2. Be familiar with the evidence from human and animal studies demonstrating sodium channel accumulation in damaged peripheral nerve and reduction in spontaneous and evoked activity in animal neuroma models.

C. Know the dosing regimens for each of these agents.

D. Be aware of the evidence from controlled trials for analgesic efficacy of intravenous lidocaine in neuropathic pain syndromes such as diabetic neuropathy and postherpetic neuralgia.

E. Be aware of the possibility for serious or irreversible toxicity with these agents (e.g., aplastic anemia from tocainide, increased risk of malignant arrhythmia from Class I antiarrhythmic agents in patients with coronary ischemia).

X. Miscellaneous adjuvant analgesics (Anthony and Lance 1969; Noyes et al. 1975; Boisen et al. 1978; Fromm 1984; Max et al. 1988; Portenoy 1990; Dellemijn and Fields 1994; Rowbotham 1994; Byas-Smith et al. 1995; Rowbotham et al. 1995)

A. Know that baclofen is proven efficacious in trigeminal neuralgia and is often used for other neuropathic lancinating pain.

B. Understand that data from controlled studies supports the efficacy of the cannabinoids as analgesics, but that toxicity limits the role of these medications.

C. Know that serotonin agonists (pizotefin, methysergide, sumatriptan), some calcium channel blockers and beta-adrenergic antagonists (e.g., propranolol) are of proven efficacy for migraine headache, but do not have evidence of analgesic activity for neuropathic or sympathetically maintained pain. Monoamine oxidase inhibitors have anecdotal evidence of efficacy in management of chronic headache.

D. Be aware of the evidence for analgesic effects of clonidine by the oral, topical, and intraspinal routes.

E. Be aware of the evidence from controlled studies for use of the topical agents capsaicin, lidocaine, and NSAIDS for neuropathic pain syndromes such as diabetic neuropathy and postherpetic neuralgia.

F. Be aware that benzodiazepines have been demonstrated in some studies to alter pain perception, but there is little evidence that they are effective analgesics for routine clinical use and are not effective compared to amitriptyline for postherpetic neuralgia.

REFERENCES

Abram, S.E. and Lightfoot, R.W., Treatment of longstanding causalgia with prazosin, Reg. Anesth., 6 (1981) 79–81.

Anthony, M. and Lance, J.W., MAO inhibition in the treatment of migraine, Arch. Neurol., 21 (1969) 263–268.

Arner, S., Intravenous phentolamine test: diagnostic and prognostic use in reflex sympathetic dystrophy, Pain, 46 (1991) 17–22.

Beaver, W.T., Wallenstein, S.L., Houde, R.W. and Rogers, A., A comparison of the analgesic effects of methotrimeprazine and morphine in patients with cancer, Clin. Pharmacol. Ther., 7 (1966) 436–446.

Bercel, N.A., Cyclobenzaprine in the treatment of skeletal muscle spasm in osteoarthritis of the cervical and lumbar spine, Curr. Ther. Res., 22 (1977) 462–468.

Blackwell, B., Side effects of antidepressant drugs, Psychiatry Update, 6 (1987) 724–725.

Boisen, E., Deth, S., Hübbe, P., Jansen, J., Klee, A. and Leunbach, G., Clonidine in the prophylaxis of migraine, Acta Neurol. Scand., 58 (1978) 288–295.

Bruera, E., Roca, E., Cedaro, L., Carraro, S. and Chacon, R., Action of oral methlprednisolone in terminal cancer patients: a prospective randomized double-blind study, Cancer Treat. Rep., 69 (1985) 751–754.

Bruera, E., Chadwick, S., Brenneis, C., Hanson, J. and MacDonald, R.N., Methylphenidate associated with narcotics for the treatment of cancer pain, Cancer Treat. Rep., 71 (1987) 67–70.

Byas-Smith, M.G., Max, M.B., Muir, J. and Kingman, A., Transdermal clonidine compared to placebo in painful diabetic neuropathy using a two-stage "enriched enrollment" design, Pain, 60 (1995) 267–274.

Carette, S., Bell, M.J., Reynolds, W.J., Haraoui, B., McCain, G.A., Bykerk, V.P., Edworthy, S.M., Baron, M., Koehler, B.E., Fam, A.G., Bellamy, N. and Guimont, C., Comparison of amitriptyline, cyclobenzaprine, and placebo in the treatment of fibromyalgia, Arthritis Rheum., 37 (1994) 32–40.

Chabal, C., Russell, L.C. and Burchiel, K.J., The effect of intravenous lidocaine, tocainide, and mexiletine on spontaneously active fibers originating in rat sciatic neuromas, Pain, 38 (1989) 333–338.

Chabal, C., Jacobson, L., Mariano, A., Chaney, E. and Britell, C.W., The use of mexiletine for the treatment of pain after peripheral nerve injury, Anesthesiology, 76 (1992) 513–517.

Couch, J.R., Ziegler, D.K. and Hassanein, R., Amitriptyline in the prophylaxis of migraine: effectiveness and relationship of antimigraine and antidepressant effects, Neurology, 26 (1976) 121–127.

Dejgard, A., Petersen, P. and Kastrup, J., Mexiletine for treatment of chronic painful diabetic neuropathy, Lancet, 1 (1988) 9–11.

Dellemijn, P.L.I. and Fields, H.L., Do benzodiazepines have a role in chronic pain management? Pain, 57 (1994) 137–152.

Dellemijn, P.L.I., Fields, H.L., Allen, R.R., McKay, W.R. and Rowbotham, M.C., The interpretation of pain relief and sensory changes following sympathetic blockade, Brain, 117 (1994) 1475–1487.

Devor, M., Govrin-Lippmann, R. and Raber, P., Corticosteroids suppress ectopic neural discharge originating in experimental neuromas, Pain, 22 (1985) 127–137.

Forrest, W.H., Brown, B., Jr., Brown, C.R., Defalque, R., Gold, M., et al., Dextroamphetamine with morphine for the treatment of postoperative pain, N. Engl. J. Med., 296 (1977) 712–715.

Fromm, G.H., Terence, C.F. and Chatta, A.S., Baclofen in the treatment of trigeminal neuralgia, Ann. Neurol., 15 (1984) 240–247.

Galer, B.S., Miller, K.V. and Rowbotham, M.C., Response to intravenous lidocaine infusion differs based on clinical diagnosis and site of nervous system injury, Neurology, 43 (1993) 1233–1235.

Ghostine, S.Y., Comair, Y.G., Turner, D.M., Kassel, N.F. and Azar, C.G., Phenoxybenzamine in the treatment of causalgia, J. Neurosurg., 60 (1984) 1263–1268.

Glassman, A.H. and Roose, S.P., Risks of antidepressants in the elderly: tricyclic antidepressants and arrhythmia-revising risks, Gerontology, 40, Suppl. 1 (1994) 15–20.

IMPACT Research Group, International mexiletine and placebo antiarrhythmic coronary trial: I. Report on arrhythmia and other findings, J. Am. Coll. Cardiol., 4 (1984) 1148–1163.

Killian, J.M. and Fromm, G.H., Carbamazepine in the treatment of neuralgia: use and side effects, Arch. Neurol., 19 (1968) 129–136.

Kozin, F., Ryan, L.M., Carerra, G.F., Soin, J.S. and Wortmann, R.L., The reflex sympathetic dystrophy syndrome (RSDS). III. Scintigraphic studies: further evidence for the therapeutic efficacy of systemic corticosteroids and proposed diagnostic criteria, Am. J. Med., 70 (1981) 23–29.

Lindstrom, P. and Lindblom, U., The analgesic effect of tocainide in rigeminal neuralgia, Pain, 28 (1987) 45–50.

Magni, G., The use of antidepressants in the treatment of chronic pain: a review of the current evidence, Drugs, 42 (1991) 730–748.

Max, M.B., Antidepressants as analgesics. In: H.L. Fields and J.C. Liebeskind (Eds.), Pharmacological Approaches to the Treatment of Chronic Pain: New Concepts and Critical Issues, Progress in Pain Research and Management, Vol. 1, IASP Press, Seattle, 1994, pp. 229–246.

Max, M., Schafer, S., Culnane, M., Smoller, B., Dubner, R. and Gracely, R.H., Amitriptyline, but not lorazepam, relieves postherpetic neuralgia, Neurology, 38 (1988) 1427–1432.

Max, M.B., Lynch, S.A., Muir, J., Shoaf, S.E., Smoller, B. and Dubner, R., Effects of desipramine, amitriptyline, and fluoxetine on pain in diabetic neuropathy, N. Engl. J. Med., 326 (1992), 1250–1256.

McQuay, H.J., Carroll, D. and Glynn, C.J., Dose-response for analgesic effect of amitriptyline in chronic pain, Anaesthesia, 48 (1993) 281–285.

Noyes, R., Brunk, S.F., Avery, D.H. and Canter, A., The analgesic properties of delta-9-tetrahydro-cannabinol and codeine, Clin. Pharmacol. Ther., 18 (1975) 84–89.

Onghena, P. and Van Houdenhove, B., Antidepressant-induced analgesia in chronic non-malignant pain: a meta-analysis of 39 placebo-controlled studies, Pain, 49 (1992) 205–220.

Portenoy, R.K., Pharmacologic management of chronic pain. Chapter 11. In: H.L. Fields (Ed.), Pain Syndromes in Neurologic Practice, Butterworths, New York, 1990, pp. 257–278.

Raja, S.N., Treede, R.D., Davis, K.D. and Campbell, J.N., Systemic alpha-adrenergic blockade with phentolamine: a diagnostic test for sympathetically maintained pain, Anesthesiology, 74 (1991) 691.

Ray, W.A., Griffin, M.R., Schaffner, W., Baugh, D.K. and Melton, L.J., Psychotropic drug use and the risk of hip fracture, N. Engl. J. Med., 316 (1987) 363–368.

Rowbotham, M.C., Topical analgesic agents. In: H.L. Fields and J.C. Liebeskind (Eds.), Pharmacological Approaches to the Treatment of Chronic Pain: New Concepts and Critical Issues, Progress in Pain Research and Management, Vol. 1, IASP Press, Seattle, 1994, pp. 211–227.

Rowbotham, M.C., Reisner, L.A. and Fields, H.L., Both intravenous lidocaine and morphine reduce the pain of post-herpetic neuralgia, Neurology, 41 (1991) 1024–1028.

Rowbotham, M.C., Davies, P.S. and Fields, H.L., Topical lidocaine gel relieves postherpetic neuralgia, Ann. Neurol., 37 (1995) 246–253.

Rumore, M.M. and Schlichting, D.A., Clinical efficacy of antihistamines as analgesics, Pain, 25 (1986) 7–22.

Sindrup, S.H., Gram, L.F., Skjold, T., Frøland, A. and Beck-Nielsen, H., Concentration-response relationship in imipramine treatment of diabetic neuropathy symptoms, Clin. Pharmacol. Ther., 47 (1990a) 509–515.

Sindrup, S.H., Gram, L.F., Brøsen, K., Eshøj, O. and Mogensen, E.F., The selective serotonin reuptake inhibitor paroxetine is effective in the treatment of diabetic neuropathy symptoms, Pain, 42 (1990b) 135–144.

Sindrup, S.H., Bjerre, U., Dejgaard, A., Brøsen, K., Aes-Jørgenson, T. and Gram, L.F., The selective serotonin reuptake inhibitor citalopram relieves the symptoms of diabetic neuropathy, Clin. Pharmacol. Ther., 52 (1992) 547–552.

Stambaugh, J.E. and Lance, C., Analgesic efficacy and pharmacokinetic evaluation of meperidine and hyroxyzine, alone and in combination, Cancer Invest., 1 (1983), 111–117.

Stracke, H., Meyer, U.E., Schumacher, H.E. and Federlin, K., Mexiletine in the treatment of diabetic neuropathy, Diabetes Care, 15 (1992) 1550–1555.

Swerdlow, M., Anticonvulsant drugs and chronic pain, Clin. Neuropharmacol., 7 (1984) 51–82.

Watson, C.P.N., Evans, R.J., Reed, K., Merskey, H. Goldsmith, L. and Warsh, J., Amitriptyline versus placebo in postherpetic neuralgia, Neurology, 32 (1982) 671–673.

Core Curriculum for Professional Education in Pain, edited by H.L. Fields, IASP Press, Seattle, © 1995.

10

Physical Medicine and Rehabilitation

I. Temperature modalities

   A. Know that heat and cold are both useful in reducing pain and spasm of musculoskeletal and neurological pathologies (Saunders 1989; Vasudevan and Hegmann 1992; Lehmann and deLateur 1994).

   B. Be aware of evidence that superficial heating of skin produces muscle relaxation due to decreased gamma fiber activity and results in decreased spindle excitability, thus decreasing pain and spasm (Fischer and Solomon 1965; Lehmann and deLateur 1994).

   C. Know that cold reduces pain, bleeding, and swelling due to vasoconstrictive properties (Kay 1985). After one or two days, heat application causes vasodilatation, which helps in healing and hematoma resolution. (Lehmann and deLateur 1978, 1994).

   D. Know that ethyl chloride spray and ice massage are counterirritants that have been used in the treatment of myofacial pain.

   E. Know that heat and cold can raise pain threshold significantly; ice therapy is more effective than heat (Benson and Copp 1974; Lehmann and deLateur 1978, 1994).

   F. Know that heat is contraindicated in acute rheumatoid arthritis and in acute trauma, as it may increase bleeding tendency and edema (Lehmann and deLateur 1994).

   G. Be aware that local temperature elevation produces many responses: increase in blood flow, increased extensibility of collagen tissues, increased capillary permeability, and enzymatic activity (Lehmann and deLateur 1978, 1994; Vasudevan 1994).

   H. Know that in short-wave diathermy, high-frequency electromagnetic current operating at frequencies of 27.12 megahertz is converted into heat, while microwave diathermy is the conversion of electromagnetic radiation in the frequencies of 2456 and 915 megahertz. Be aware that short-wave diathermy and microwave diathermy selectively heat muscles (Michlovitz 1986).

   I. Be aware that ultrasound is high-frequency vibration at .8–1 megahertz, which is converted into heat. Ultrasound selectively heats muscles, tendons, and tendon-bone junctions (Lehmann and deLateur 1978, 1994).

   J. Know that superficial heat includes hot packs, heating pads, paraffin wax, fluidotherapy, hydrotherapy, Hubbard tank, whirlpool, and radiant heat (heat lamps). Superficial heat produces heating of only the superficial tissues up to .5 cm from the surface of the skin, while deep heating modalities heat to the depth of 3–5 cm (Michlovitz 1986; Vasudevan and Hegmann 1992).

K. Know that in ice massage a block of ice is rubbed over the skin surface. The initial phase of cooling is followed in 2–3 minutes by a period of burning, followed by analgesia (Michlovitz 1986; Vasudevan and Hegmann 1992; Vasudevan 1994).

L. Know that temperature modalities should rarely be used alone, but in conjunction with appropriate exercises such as stretching for range of motion and for strengthening after pain reduction (Vasudevan and Hegmann 1992; Vasudevan 1994).

M. Heating modalities should not be used for patients with impaired consciousness, over anesthetized areas, where circulation is decreased over active malignancies, or over gonads or a developing fetus (Lehmann and deLateur 1978, 1994).

N. Know that short-wave diathermy and microwave diathermy are contraindicated in the presence of metal implants and cardiac pacemakers. Those heating modalities selectively heat metal and may interfere with some cardiac pacemakers. Ultrasound is contraindicated over areas containing fluid, such as the eyes, over amniotic fluid in pregnant women, and over joints with active effusion (Lehmann and deLateur 1978; Michlovitz 1986; Lehmann and deLateur 1994).

II. Manipulation, mobilization, massage, and traction

A. Be aware that massage and mobilization are widely used for treating pain problems, especially back pain (Basmajian 1985; Haldemann 1992, 1994).

B. Know that spinal and peripheral joint mobilization and manipulation are frequently used to treat pain. Be aware of the difference between joint mobilization and manipulation (Haldemann 1994; Wood 1974).

C. Be aware that massage is the application of touch or force to soft tissues, usually muscles, tendons, or ligaments, without causing movement or change of joint position (Wood 1974; Rogoff 1981).

D. Know that massage includes several types and techniques:

1. Stroking or effleurage, which involves light movement of the hands over the skin in a slow, rhythmic fashion (Rogoff 1981)
2. Kneading massage or pétrissage, which involves deep handling of tissues in preparation for stretching of muscles (Rogoff 1981)
3. Tapotement is the use of percussion, clapping, shaking, and vibrations (Cyriax 1971; Hofkosh 1983; Wood 1974).

E. Understand that mobilization includes those procedures in which a therapist uses hands and fingers to handle tissues. The mobilization is used to increase range of motion beyond the resistance that limits passive range of motion or exercises. Mobilization differs from manipulation or adjustment in that there is no forceful thrust or jerking motion (Haldemann 1994).

F. Sustained progressive stretching is included in stretch and spray technique to inactivate triggers points. This technique involves stretching tight muscles with active trigger points while the overlying skin is sprayed with a vapo coolant such as ethylchloride or fluoromethane (Mennell 1960; Haldemann 1992).

G. Spinal adjustment or manipulation involves small-amplitude and high-velocity thrusts. This action is thought to correct the misalignment and increase the range of spinal motion (Nwuga 1982; Haldemann 1992, 1994).

H. Be aware that despite patient satisfaction and acceptance of massage treatment, there are no controlled studies to show its effectiveness (Haldemann 1994).

I. Although controversial, there is evidence that manipulation hastens recovery from acute, uncomplicated, low back pain (Shekelle et al. 1992; Haldemann 1994).

J. Traction is a mechanical distraction of tissues, done manually or mechanically. It is an adjunct in treatment of soft tissue problems. Overhead cervical traction is one of the effective techniques for the treatment of cervical radiculopathy (Vasudevan 1994).

III. Exercises

A. Know the purpose of using exercises in the management of pain.

B. Be aware that exercise programs may be useful for both acute and chronic pain problems. Understand the specific use to maintain muscle strength, range of motion, and general conditioning with various pain problems (Sullivan and Markos 1987; Linton 1994).

C. Know that immobilization can reduce strength and function of muscles, ligaments, and tendons. Prescribed exercises that increase the forces being transmitted to muscles, ligaments, tendons, and bones will maintain and gradually increase the strength and functional capacity of these structures (Tipton et al. 1986).

D. Understand that the goals of therapeutic exercises include: increased strength, endurance, range of motion, coordination, and balance to reduce pain, spasm, edema, and postural deviations (Wells and Lessard 1994).

E. Know that exercises include passive, active assistive, active, resistive, progressive resistive, and stretching exercises. Relaxation and general aerobic conditioning exercises increase cardiovascular endurance (Vasudevan and Hegmann 1992).

F. Passive movements reduce pain and stiffness and improve function (Strickland and Glogovac 1980; Farrell 1985; Saunders 1989).

G. Know that there is evidence that patients with herniated nucleus pulposus with low back and leg pain can benefit from an aggressive physical exercise program (Saal 1990).

H. Know that stretching exercises are important for muscles that cross two joints—hamstrings, gastrocnemius, hip flexors, pectoral, and paraspinal muscles. Stretching should be done slowly and steadily, while avoiding bouncing and jerking activities.

I. Be aware that aerobic exercises to increase cardiopulmonary capacity, fitness, and endurance include rhythmic, repetitive, dynamic activities, such as running, cycling, and swimming. These activities involve large muscle groups and should be preceded and followed by stretching exercises. There is evidence that stretching exercises and aerobic conditioning exercises can help some patients with chronic pain of musculoskeletal origin.

REFERENCES

Basmajian, J.V., Manipulation, Traction and Massage, 3rd ed., Williams & Wilkins, Baltimore, 1985.

Benson, T.B. and Copp, E.P., The effects of therapeutic forms of heat and ice on pain threshold of normal shoulder, Rheumatology and Rehabilitation, 13 (1974) 101–104.

Boyling, J.F., Ergonomics and management of pain. In: P.E. Wells, V. Frampton and D. Bowsher, (Eds.), Pain Management by Physical Therapy, 2nd ed., Butterworth-Heinemann, Oxford, 1994, pp. 29–38.

Cyriax, E.T., Textbook of Orthopedic Medicine: Diagnosis of Soft Tissue Lesions, Vol. 1, 6th ed., Bailiere Tindall, London, 1971.

deLateur, B.J. and Lehmann, J.F., Strengthening exercises. In: J.K. Leek, M.E. Gershwin and W.M. Fowler (Eds.), Principles of Physical Medicine and Rehabilitation in Musculoskeletal Diseases, Grune & Stratton, Orlando, 1986.

Farrell, P.A., Exercises and endorphins: male response, Med. Sci. Sports Exerc., 17 (1985) 89–93.

Fields, H.L. and Basbaum, A.I., Brainstem control of spinal pain - transmission neurons, Ann. Rev. Physiol., 40 (1985) 217–248.

Fischer, E. and Solomon, S., Physiological responses to heat and cold. In: S. Licht (Ed.), Therapeutic Heat and Cold, 2nd ed., Waverly Press, Baltimore, 1965.

Grabois, M., Treatment of pain syndromes through exercise. In: D.T. Lowenthal, K. Bharadwaja and W.W. Oaks (Eds.), Therapeutics Through Exercise, Grune & Stratton, New York, 1979.

Haldemann, S., Principles and Practice of Chiropractic, Appelton & Lange, Norwalk, 1992.

Haldemann, S., Manipulation and massage for the relief of back pain. In: Textbook of Pain, P.D. Wall and R. Melzack (Eds.), Vol. 3, Churchill-Livingstone, Edinburgh, 1994, pp. 1251–1262.

Hofkosh, J.M., Clinical massage. In: J.V. Basmajian (Ed.), Manipulation, Traction and Massage, 3rd ed., Williams & Wilkins, Baltimore, 1983.

Jackson, C. and Bro, M., Is there a role for exercises in the treatment of patients with low back pain? Clin. Orthop., 179 (1983) 39–43.

Kaplan, P.E. and Tanner, E.D., Musculoskeletal Pain and Disability, Appleton & Lange, Norwalk, 1989.

Kay, D.B., Sprained ankle: current therapy, Foot Ankle, 6 (1985) 22–28.

Kessler, R.M. and Herling, D., Management of Common Musculoskeletal Disorders: Physical Therapies, Principles and Method, Harper & Row, New York, 1983.

King, J.C., Dumitru, D. and Walsh, E., Rehabilitation of the pain patients: a US perspective, Pain Digest, 2 (1992) 106–126.

Leek, J.C., Gershwin, M.E. and Fowler, W.M., Principles of Physical Medicine and Rehabilitation in Musculoskeletal Disease, Grun & Stratton, Gaavanovich Publication, New York, 1986.

Lehmann, J.F. and deLateur, B.J., Therapeutic heat. In: P.D. Wall and R. Melzack (Eds.), Textbook of Pain, Churchill Livingstone, Edinburgh, 1984.

Lehmann, J.F. and deLateur, B.J., Ultrasound, shortwave, microwave, laser, superficial heat and cold in the treatment of pain, In: P.D. Wall and R. Melzack, (Eds.), Textbook of Pain, 1994; 3rd ed, Churchill-Livingstone, Edinburgh, 1994, pp. 1237–1248.

Linton, S.J., The challenge of preventing musculoskeletal pain. In: G.B. Gebhart, D.L. Hammond and T.S. Jensen (Eds.), Proceedings of 7th World Congress on Pain, Progress in Pain Research and Management, Vol. 2, IASP Press, Seattle, 1994, pp. 149–166.

Low, J., Electrotherapeutic modalities. In: P.E. Wells, V. Frampton and D. Bowsher (Eds.), Pain Management by Physical Therapy, 2nd. ed., Butterworth-Heinemann, Oxford, 1994, pp. 140–176.

Maitland, G.D., Vertebral Manipulation, 3rd ed., Butterworth, London, 1973.

Michlovitz, S., Thermal Agents in Rehabilitation, F.A. Davis, Philadelphia, 1986.

Mayer, T., Gatchel, R., Mayer, H., Kishino, N., Keeley, J. and Mooney, V., A prospective two-year study of functional restoration in industrial low back injury: an objective assessment procedure, JAMA, 258 (1987) 1763–1767.

Mennell, J.B., Back Pain: Diagnosis and Treatment Using Manipulative Therapy, Little, Brown and Co., Boston, 1960.

Nwuga, V.C.B., A relative therapeutic efficacy of vertebral manipulations and conventional treatment in back pain management, Am. J. Phys. Med. Rehabil., 61 (1982) 273–278.

Rogoff, J.B., (Ed.), Manipulation, Traction and Massage, Williams & Wilkins, Baltimore, 1981.

Saal, S.R., Dynamic muscular stabilization in the non-operative treatment of lumbar pain syndromes, Orthop. Rev., 19 (1990) 691–699.

Saunders, S.R., Physical therapy of hand fractures, Phys. Ther., 69 (1989) 1065–1076.

Shekelle, B.G., Adams, A.H., Chassin, M.R., Hurwitz, E.C. and Brook, R.H., Spinal manipulation for low back pain, Ann. Intern. Med., 117 (1992) 590–598.

Strickland, J.W. and Glogovac, S.V., Digital function following flexure tendon repair in zone II: a comparison of immobilization and controlled passive motion techniques, J. Hand Surg., 5 (1980) 537–543.

Sullivan, P.E. and Markos, P.D., Clinical Procedures in Therapeutic Exercises, Appleton & Lange, Norwalk, 1987.

Tipton, C.M., Vailas, A.C. and Matthess, R.D., Experimental studies on the influence of physical activity on ligaments, tendons, and joints: a brief review, Acta Medica Scandinavia (Suppl.), 710 (1986) 157–168.

Travell, J.G. and Simons, D.G. (Eds.), Myofacial Pain and Dysfunction: The Trigger Point Manual, Williams & Wilkins, Baltimore, 1983.

Travell, J.G., Myofacial trigger points: clinical view, Advances in Pain and Research Therapy, 1 (1976) 919–926.

Unruh, A., Baster, D.G. and Casale, R., Pain curriculum for students in occupational therapy or physical therapy, IASP Newsletter, Nov./Dec. 1994, pp. 3–8.

Vasudevan, S.V., Physical rehabilitation of the pain patient. In: P.P. Raj (Ed.), Current Review of Pain, Current Medicine, Philadelphia, 1994, pp. 130–140.

Vasudevan, S.V., Hegmann, K., Moore, A. and Cerletty, S., Physical methods of pain management. In: P.P. Raj (Ed.), Practical Management of Pain, 2nd ed., Yearbook Medical Publishers, Chicago, 1992, pp. 669–679.

Wells, P.E., Manipulative procedures. In: P.E. Wells, V. Frampton and D. Bowsher (Eds.), Pain Management by Physical Therapy, 2nd ed., Butterworth-Heinemann, Oxford, 1994, pp. 187–212.

Wells, P. and Lessard, E., Movement education and limitations of movement. In: P. Wall and R. Melzack (Eds.), Textbook of Pain, 2nd ed., Churchill-Livingstone, Edinburgh, 1994, pp. 1263–1276.

Wood, E.C., Beard's Massage: Principles and Techniques, W.B. Saunders, Philadelphia, 1974.

Core Curriculum for Professional Education in Pain, edited by H.L. Fields, IASP Press, Seattle, © 1995.

11

Nonsurgical Peripherally Applied Neuroaugmentative and Counterirritation Techniques

I. Know different peripheral stimulation techniques used to produce analgesia.

  A. Transcutaneous electrical nerve stimulation (TENS) (Woolf and Thompson 1994)
  B. Acupuncture-like TENS or hyperstimulation (Melzack 1994)
  C. Vibration (Lundeberg et al. 1987)
  D. Acupuncture, dry needling, or electro-acupuncture (Firebrace and Hill 1994)

II. Understand the postulated mechanisms of peripheral stimulation-induced analgesia.

  A. Segmental

    1. Selective activation of large, low-threshold A-beta afferent fibers produces a spatially restricted pre- and postsynaptic inhibition of dorsal horn neurons reducing nociceptive afferent evoked responses (Woolf and Thompson 1994).
    2. Know about gamma aminobutyric acid (GABA), glycine, and inhibitory interneurons in the substantia gelatinosa.
    3. Know the historical contribution of the spinal gate-control theory (Melzack and Wall 1965).

  B. Extrasegmental

    1. Stimulation of small-caliber high-threshold A-delta and C nociceptive fibers produces a generalized inhibition of dorsal horn neurons that arises primarily by activation of descending inhibitory pathways from the brain stem (Fields and Basbaum 1994).
    2. Know about the diffuse noxious inhibitory control model, on/off cells in the medulla, and the synaptic pharmacology of descending inhibition (Fields and Basbaum 1994).

  C. Cortical

    1. High-level cognitive/emotional inputs initiate poorly understood mechanisms at different levels of the neuraxis to control nociceptive sensory processing.
    2. Know that this is likely to contribute to efficacy of suggestion, placebo, and many folk medicine therapies.

  D. Peripheral

    1. Limited evidence suggests that peripheral stimulation alters blood blow and peripheral chemicals (Kaada 1985; Kashiba and Yoshihiro 1991).

III. Be aware of the parameters of stimulation.

    A. Conventional TENS

        1. Generally high frequency (50–100 Hz) and low intensity (paresthesia but not painful); The stimulation parameters giving the best results need to be evaluated for each patient (Johnson et al. 1991; Woolf and Thompson 1994).

        2. A stimulation duration of 30 minutes is sufficient for a significant reduction of both experimental and clinical pain. However, advantages of longer stimulation have been suggested (Wynn Parry 1980; Woolf 1989; Marchand et al. 1993).

        3. Electrode localization: paresthesia must cover the painful region (Ottoson and Lundeberg 1988; Johnson et al. 1991).

        4. Pulse width: between 50 and 200 µs. Longer pulses may be required for deep pain.

    B. Acupuncture-like TENS or hyperstimulation

        1. Low-frequency (2–10 Hz), high-intensity (to tolerance threshold) stimuli or brief trains of high-frequency (100–200 Hz) stimuli repeated at low frequency. The higher intensities (near pain tolerance) produce the best results (Melzack 1975).

        2. Duration: about 30 minutes

        3. Localization: the stimulation usually should not overlap the painful area, but a trial-and-error approach is required to optimize efficacy

        4. Pulse width: as for TENS, pulse width between 50 and 200 µs

    C. Vibration

        1. Electromechanical, high frequency (100–200 Hz) and low intensity (strong but not painful) (Ekblom and Hansson 1982; Lundeberg et al. 1987)

        2. Duration: 30–45 minutes

        3. Localization: over the painful area (Lundeberg et al. 1987)

    D. Acupuncture, dry needling

        1. For dry needling, several different manipulations of the needles are used including rotation, electrical stimulation, or multiple insertion (Xi et al. 1992; Firebrace and Hill 1994).

        2. Duration: variable

        3. Localization: traditional Chinese acupuncture points. Some studies find no difference between real and false points, while others find an advantage to using the real points. Insertion of needles at trigger points is effective for treatment of musculoskeletal or myofascial pains (Gaw et al. 1975; Tauh et al. 1977; Brockhaus and Elger 1990; Bernfield and Karngold 1992).

IV. Be familiar with the clinical applications of neuroaugmentative therapies.

    A. Conventional TENS or vibration

        1. TENS reduces pain in different acute and chronic pain conditions including low back pain, deafferentation pain, causalgia, pain during delivery, acute orofacial pain, and acute and chronic arthritic pain (Meyer and Fields 1972; Mannheimer and Carlsson 1979; Hansson and Ekblom 1983; Roche et al. 1984; Davies 1989; Leandri et al. 1990; Marchand et al. 1993).

2. The analgesic effect of TENS is generally not sufficient to manage for intense acute pain such as in dental surgery but can reduce anesthetic requirement during surgery (Bourke et al. 1984; Hansson and Ekblom 1984).

3. Similar results are reported for vibration analgesia (Lundeberg et al. 1987; Ter Riet et al. 1990; Guieu et al. 1991).

4. Even if analgesic effects of TENS are generally reported as brief and fading over time, some long-term benefits are reported, for some patients (Johnson et al. 1991).

B. Acupuncture-like TENS or hyperstimulation

1. As for TENS, hyperstimulation has been successfully used for different chronic and acute pain conditions, but its painful character limits patients' acceptance (Melzack 1994).

2. The diffuse quality of hyperstimulation may be useful in some pain conditions where the stimulation can not be applied to the painful site.

C. Acupuncture

1. As for TENS and vibration, several studies report good results with acupuncture for different pain conditions. However, a meta-analysis of the literature reveals highly contradictory results. Most clinical trials are poorly designed. Efficacy is still debatable (Ter Riet et al. 1990; Xi et al. 1992; Thomas and Lundberg 1994).

2. The neurobiological rationale for this type of treatment is still poorly understood.

V. Efficacy

A. Know that the results of treatment are variable in clinical and experimental studies. Be aware that no clear criteria have been identified to decide if a patient will benefit or not from neuroaugmentative treatment.

B. Understand that the analgesic effect of TENS may be potentiated by repetitive use and that the efficacy of treatment may improve over time (Johnson et al. 1991; Marchand et al. 1993).

C. Know that even if suggestibility and predisposition of the patients are important contributors, TENS and vibration are better than placebo in some studies but that failures are common (Conn et al. 1986; Harrison et al. 1986; Lundeberg et al. 1987; Marchand et al. 1993). Be aware of the difficulty in designing placebo treatments to compare with neuroaugmentative therapy (Marchand et al. 1993).

D. Be aware of the relatively short duration of the effects and habituation over time.

REFERENCES

Bernfield, H. and Karngold, E., Between Heaven and Earth: A Guide to Chinese Medicine, Ballantine, New York, 1992.

Bourke, D.L., Smith, B.A., Erickson, J., Gwartz, B. and Lessard, L., TENS reduces halothane requirement during hand surgery, Anesthesiology, 61 (1984) 769–722.

Brockhaus, A. and Elger, C.E., Hypalgesic efficacy of acupuncture on experimental pain in man: comparison of laser acupuncture and needle acupuncture, Pain, 43 (1990) 181–185.

Conn, I.G., Marshall, A.H., Yadav, S.N., Daly, J.C. and Jaffer, M., Transcutaneous electrical nerve stimulation following appendectomy: the placebo effect, Ann. R. Coll. Surg. Engl., 68 (1986) 191–192.

Davies, P., An evaluation of transcutaneous nerve stimulation for the relief of pain in labour, J. Assoc. Chart. Physiother. Obstet. Gynaecol., 65 (1989) 2–7.

Ekblom, A. and Hansson, P., Effects of conditioning vibratory stimuli on pain threshold of the human tooth, Acta. Physiol. Scand., 114 (1982) 601–604.

Fields, H.L. and Basbaum, A.I., Central nervous system mechanisms of pain modulation. In: P.D. Wall and R. Melzack (Eds.), The Textbook of Pain, 3rd ed., Churchill Livingstone, Edinburgh, 1994, pp. 243–257.

Firebrace, P. and Hill, S., Acupuncture: How It Works, How It Cures, Keats Publishing, New Canaan, 1994.

Gaw, A.C., Chang, L.W. and Shaw, L.-C., Efficacy of acupuncture on osteoarthritic pain, N. Engl. J. Med., 293 (1975) 375–378.

Guieu, R., Tardy-Gervet, M.-F. and Roll, J.-P., Analgesic effects of vibration and transcutaneous electrical nerve stimulation applied separately and simultaneously to patients with chronic pain, Can. J. Neurol. Sci., 18 (1991) 113–119.

Hansson, P. and Ekblom, A., Transcutaneous electrical nerve stimulation (TENS) as compared to placebo TENS for the relief of acute oro-facial pain, Pain, 15 (1983) 157–165.

Hansson, P. and Ekblom, A., Afferent stimulation induced pain relief in acute oro-facial pain and its failure to induce sufficient pain reduction in dental and oral surgery, Pain, 20 (1984) 273–278.

Harrison, R.F., Woods, T., Shore, M., Mathews, G. and Unwin, A., Pain relief in labour using transcutaneous electrical nerve stimulation (TENS). A TENS/TENS placebo controlled study in two parity groups, Br. J. Obstet. Gynaecol., 93 (1986) 739–746.

Johnson, M.I., Ashton, C.H. and Thompson, J.W., An in-depth study of long-term users of transcutaneous electrical nerve stimulation (TENS): implications for clinical use of TENS, Pain, 44 (1991) 221–229.

Kaada, B., Mechanisms of vasodilatation evoked by transcutaneous nerve stimulation, Acupunct. Electrother. Res., 10 (1985) 217–219.

Kashiba, H. and Yoshihiro, U., Acupuncture to the skin induced release of substance P and calcitonin gene-related peptide from peripheral terminals of primary sensory neurons in the rat, Am. J. Chin. Med., 3-4 (1991) 189–197.

Leandri, M., Parodi, C.I., Corrieri, N. and Rigardo, S., Comparison of TENS treatments in hemiplegic shoulder pain, Scand. J. Rehabil. Med., 22 (1990) 69–72.

Lundeberg, T., Abrahamsson, P., Bondesson, L. and Haker, E., Vibratory stimulation compared to placebo in alleviation of pain, Scand. J. Rehabil. Med., 19 (1987) 153–158.

Mannheimer, C. and Carlsson, C.-A., The analgesic effect of transcutaneous electrical nerve stimulation (TENS) in patients with rheumatoid arthritis: a comparative study of different pulse patterns, Pain, 6 (1979) 329–334.

Marchand, S., Charest, J., Li, J., Chenard, J.-R., Lavignolle, B. and Laurencelle, L., Is TENS purely a placebo effect? A controlled study on low back pain, Pain, 54 (1993) 99–106.

Melzack, R., Prolonged relief of pain by brief, intense transcutaneous somatic stimulation, Pain, 1 (1975) 357–373.

Melzack, R., Folk medicine and the sensory modulation of pain. In: P.D. Wall and R. Melzack (Eds.), Textbook of Pain, 3rd ed., Churchill Livingstone, Edinburgh, 1994, pp. 897–905.

Melzack, R. and Wall, P.D., Pain mechanisms: a new theory, Science, 150 (1965) 971–979.

Meyer, G.A. and Fields, H.L., Causalgia treated by selective large fibre stimulation of peripheral nerve, Brain, 95 (1972) 163–168.

Ottoson, D. and Lundeberg, T., Pain Treatment by Transcutaneous Electrical Nerve Stimulation: A Practical Manual, Springer-Verlag, New York, 1988.

Roche, P.A., Gijsbers, K., Belch, J.J.F. and Forbes, C.D., Modification of haemophilic haemorrhage pain by transcutaneous electrical nerve stimulation, Pain, 21 (1984) 43–48.

Tauh, H.A., Beard, M.C., Eisenberg, L. and McCormack, R.K., Studies of acupuncture for operative dentistry, Journal of Acupuncture and Operative Dentistry, 95 (1977) 55–61.

Ter Riet, G., Kleijnen, J. and Knipschild, P., Acupuncture and chronic pain: a criteria-based meta-analysis, J. Clin. Epidemiol., 43 (1990) 1191–1199.

Thomas, M. and Lundberg, T., Importance of modes of acupuncture in the treatment of chronic nociceptive low back pain, Acta Anaesthesiol. Scand., 38 (1994) 63–69.

Woolf, C.J., Afferent induced alterations of receptive field properties. In: F. Cervero, G.J. Bennett and P.M. Headley (Eds.), Processing of Sensory Information in the Superficial Dorsal Horn of the Spinal Cord, Plenum NATO ASI Series, New York, 1989, pp. 443–462.

Woolf, C.J. and Thompson, S.W.N., Segmental afferent fibre induced analgesia: transutaneous electrical nerve stimulation and vibration. In: P.D. Wall and R. Melzack (Eds.), Textbook of Pain, 3rd ed., Churchill Livingston, Edinburgh, 1994, pp. 884–896.

Wynn Parry, C.B., Pain in avulsion lesions of the brachial plexus, Pain, 9 (1980) 41–53.

Xi, D., Han, J., Zhang, Z. and Sun, Z., Acupuncture treatment of rheumatoid arthritis and exploration of acupuncture manipulations, J. Tradit. Chin. Med., 12 (1992) 35–40.

Core Curriculum for Professional Education in Pain, edited by H.L. Fields, IASP Press, Seattle, © 1995.

12

Surgical Approaches

I. Introduction and indications (White and Sweet 1969; Willis 1985; Tasker 1987; Gybels and Sweet 1989; Tasker and Dostrovsky 1989)

   A. Know the general health issues that are relevant to a successful surgical procedure.

   B. Know the importance of the following in evaluating a patient for surgery:

      1. Disease-causing pain
      2. Life expectancy
      3. Adequate trial of nonsurgical management, particularly for those drugs that are known to be effective in selected pain disorders
      4. Cancer versus noncancer pain including the role of cancer in neural injury pain
      5. Pain due to injury to the nervous system
      6. Role of nerve blocks in patient evaluation
      7. Identification and assessment of psychological and environmental factors influencing pain behavior
      8. Patient's, family's, and referring physician's expectations of surgical treatment

II. Specific procedures: indications, techniques, outcome

   A. General (Tasker and Dostrovsky 1989; Tasker 1994b)

      1. Be aware of the complications of destructive surgery to relieve pain and of the prevalence of pain recurrence.
      2. Be aware of the advantages and disadvantages of percutaneous versus open approaches for destructive surgery.

   B. Peripheral neurectomy (White and Sweet 1969; Aids to the Examination . . . 1986; Tasker 1987; Gybels and Sweet 1989; Tasker and Dostrovsky 1989; Wood 1989; Loeser et al. 1990; Bennett 1994; Loeser 1994).

      1. Know the limited utility of peripheral neurectomy in pain management including the treatment of tic douloureux.
      2. Be aware of proposed mechanisms for pain caused by injury to the nervous system including iatrogenic injuries, and the role of neuromas (Chapter 20).
      3. Understand the unique features of tic douloureux which usually affects the trigeminal but occasionally the IXth–Xth cranial nerves.

   C. Sympathectomy (Gybels and Sweet 1989, p. 257; Tasker and Lougheed 1990; Bennett 1994; Hardy and Bay 1995)

    1. Know the indications for sympathectomy for pain relief.

        a. Pain of vascular origin
        b. Visceral pain

    2. Know how to evaluate a patient by tests of sympathetic function and by use of local or regional anesthesia.
    3. Know available techniques and outcome data.

D. For spinal dorsal rhizotomy including ganglionectomy (Gybels and Sweet 1989, p. 109; Wood 1989; Dubuisson 1994; Taub et al. 1995)

    1. Know the indications.

        a. Cancer
        b. Occipital neuralgia, intercostal neuralgia, sciatica

    2. Be aware of the various techniques, open and percutaneous.
    3. Know how to interpret the results of nerve blocks in planning spinal dorsal rhizotomy.
    4. Know the expected outcomes.

E. Anterolateral spinal tractotomy (cordotomy) (White and Sweet 1969; Willis 1985; Lipton 1989; Sweet and Poletti 1994; Tasker 1995)

    1. Indications: cancer pain
    2. Know the available techniques, open and percutaneous
    3. Understand their relative outcomes with respect to:

        a. Pain recurrence
        b. Complications
        c. The pathophysiology of respiratory difficulties

F. The dorsal root entry zone (DREZ) procedures, spinal and medullary (Nashold et al. 1995)

    1. Know the indications.

        a. Brachial plexus avulsion
        b. Postherpetic neuralgia

    2. Be aware of the techniques.
    3. Know the outcome data.

G. Commissural myelotomy (Gybels and Sweet 1989; Sweet and Poletti 1994)

    1. Know that the major indication is midline cancer pain in the pelvic area.
    2. Be aware of the techniques:

        a. Open
        b. Percutaneous

    3. Recognize that pain relief may not be restricted to the region of hypalgesia or the somatotopy of the area lesioned.

H. Facet rhizolysis (Bogduk 1988; North et al. 1994)

    1. Know the indications.
    2. Understand the innervation of the facet joints.
    3. Know how to evaluate diagnostic nerve blocks.
    4. Be aware of the different techniques under local and general anesthesia with and without physiological localization.
    5. Be aware of outcome data.

I. Operations on the cranial nerve roots (Jannetta et al. 1990; Sweet 1990; Loeser 1994; Linderoth and Håkanson 1995; Sweet and Poletti 1995)

    1. Know the indications for:

        a. Tic douloureux (V, IX–X)
            (1) Understand how to diagnose tic.
            (2) Know the techniques available for tic:
                (a) Percutaneous RF rhizolysis
                (b) Percutaneous glycerol injection
                (c) Microcompression
                (d) Microvascular decompression
                (e) Open V rhizotomy in posterior fossa
                (f) Open IX–X rhizotomy
        b. Cancer (rarely): percutaneous RF rhizolysis

    2. Be aware of the expected outcomes.

J. Destructive procedures on the brain and brainstem (White and Sweet 1969; Willis 1985; Frank et al. 1987; Gybels and Sweet 1989; Jannetta et al. 1990; Bouckoms 1994; Sweet and Poletti 1994; Tasker 1994a; Ballantine et al. 1995)

    1. Appreciate that the stereotactic approach is probably the chief technique by which such procedures are accomplished with the exception of cingulumotomy.
    2. Understand the basic principles of stereotaxis: use of frames, imaging, computer assistance, physiology and (usually) RF lesion-making.
    3. Know that cancer pain is the major indication for these procedures.
    4. Be aware of the procedures currently in use.

        a. Stereotactic mesencephalic tractotomy
        b. Stereotactic medial thalamotomy
        c. Stereotactic or free-hand percutaneous radiofrequency cingulumotomy

    5. Be aware of anecdotal nature of the outcome data.

K. Hypophysectomy (Miles 1994)

    1. Know that cancer pain is the major indication.
    2. Be aware of the techniques.

        a. Be aware of historical approaches: open, subfrontal, transphenoidal.
        b. Stereotactic

    c. Free-hand percutaneous

    d. Be aware of the different methods used historically for lesion-making: ablative, radioactive sources, radiofrequency; alcohol injection currently is the most common.

  3. Be aware of outcome data for transphenoidal alcohol injection.

L. Neurostimulation techniques (Willis 1985; Levy et al. 1987; Meyerson 1990; Young and Rinaldi 1994; North 1995)

  1. Be aware of:

    a. The historical development of neurostimulation techniques

    b. The general principles of stimulation techniques

      (1) Safety principles in the use of chronic stimulation

      (2) The role of test stimulation

      (3) The need to produce paresthesiae in the area of pain

      (4) Follow-up and management of the patient with an implanted stimulator

      (5) Troubleshooting a defective stimulator

      (6) Be aware of the proposed pathophysiological principles thought to be at work in chronic stimulation for the relief of pain.

  2. Peripheral nerve stimulation, know the:

    a. Indications: neuropathic pain

    b. Techniques and equipment available

    c. Outcome data

  3. Spinal cord stimulation

    a. Know the indications.

      (1) Neuropathic pain

      (2) Pain of degenerative disc disease

        (a) Leg pain

        (b) Possibly low back pain

    b. Know the cord stimulation sites for treating pain in different parts of the body.

    c. Techniques

      (1) Open with insertion of plate-type electrodes

      (2) Percutaneous: be aware of the different electrode arrays available and their proposed indications.

      (3) Be aware of the two basic methods of chronic stimulation: radiofrequency-coupled and totally implantable and programmable.

  4. Deep brain stimulation (DBS)

    a. Be aware that there are two basic DBS techniques, paresthesiae-producing and medial stimulation.

    b. Be aware of the suggested rationale for each.

    c. Know the indications.

      (1) Neuropathic pain

      (2) "Failed back" pain

      (3) Cancer and other nociceptive pain

    d. Be aware of the equipment available (similar to that for dorsal column stimulation).

    e. Be aware of outcome data.

M. Epidural spinal and intrathecal opioid administration (Cousins and Mather 1984; Lazorthes et al. 1988; Gybels and Sweet 1989, p 319; Portenoy 1991; Lenzi et al. 1995)

1. Know the indications.

    a. Cancer pain

    b. Understand the current controversy regarding use in non-cancer pain.

2. Understand the physiological basis (Chapter 5).

3. Know how to use test-dosing.

4. Be aware of techniques available.

    a. Intraspinal:
      (1) Epidural
      (2) Intrathecal

    b. Intraventricular

5. Understand determination of dosage of morphine and its continued administration, the management of the equipment and how to troubleshoot problems.

6. Understand outcome data.

REFERENCES

Aids to the Examination of the Peripheral Nervous System, Bailliere Tindall, London, 1986.

Ballantine, H.T., Jr., Cosgrove, G.R. and Giriunas, I.E., Surgical treatment of intractable psychiatric illness and chronic pain by stereotactic cingulotomy. In: H.H. Schmidek and W.H. Sweet (Eds.), Operative Neurosurgical Techniques, 3rd ed., Saunders, Philadelphia, 1995, pp. 1423–1430.

Bennett, G.J., Neuropathic pain. In: P.D. Wall and R. Melzack (Eds.), Textbook of Pain, 3rd ed., Churchill Livingstone, Edinburgh, 1994, pp. 201–224.

Bogduk, N., Back pain: zygapophysial blocks and epidural steroids. In: M.J. Cousins and P.O. Bridenbaugh (Eds.), Neural Blockade in Clinical Anesthesia and Management of Pain, 2nd ed., Lippincott, Philadelphia, 1988, pp. 935–954.

Bouckoms, A.J., Psychosurgery for pain. In: P.D. Wall and R. Melzack (Eds.), Textbook of Pain, 3rd ed., Churchill Livingstone, Edinburgh, 1994, pp. 1171–1187.

Cousins, M.J. and Mather, L.E., Intrathecal and epidural administration of opioids, Anesthesiology, 61 (1984) 276–310.

Dubuisson, D., Root surgery. In: P.D. Wall and R. Melzack (Eds.), Textbook of Pain, 3rd ed., Churchill Livingstone, Edinburgh, 1994, pp. 1055–1065.

Frank, F., Fabrizi, A.P., Gaist, G., Weigel, K. and Mundinger, F., Stereotactic lesions in the treatment of chronic cancer pain syndromes: mesencephalotomy versus multiple thalamotomies, Applied Neurophysiology, 50 (1987) 314–318.

Gybels, J.M. and Sweet, W.H., Neurosurgical Treatment of Persistent Pain, Karger, Basel, 1989.

Hardy, R.W. and Bay, J.W., Surgery of the sympathetic nervous system. In: H.H. Schmidek and W.H. Sweet (Eds.), Operative Neurosurgical Techniques, 3rd ed., Saunders, Philadelphia, 1995, pp. 1637–1646.

Jannetta, P.J., Gildenberg, P.L., Loeser, J.D., Sweet, W.H. and Ojemann, G.A., Operations on the brain and brainstem for chronic pain. In: J.J. Bonica (Ed.), The Management of Pain, 2nd ed., Febiger, Philadelphia, 1990, pp. 2082–2103.

Lazorthes, Y., Verdie, J.-C., Caute, B., Maranhao, R. and Jafani, M., Intracerebroventricular morphinotherapy for control of chronic cancer pain. In: H.L. Fields and J.M. Besson (Eds.), Pain Modulation, Progress in Brain Research, Vol. 77, Elsevier Science Publishers, Amsterdam, 1988, pp. 395–405.

Lenzi, A., Galli, G. and Marini, G., Intraventricular morphine in the treatment of pain secondary to cancer. In: H.H. Schmidek and W.H. Sweet (Eds.), Operative Neurosurgical Techniques, 3rd ed., Saunders, Philadelphia, 1995, pp. 1431–1441.

Levy, R.M., Lamb, S. and Adams, J.E., Treatment of chronic pain by deep brain stimulation: long term follow-up and review of the literature, Neurosurgery, 21 (1987) 885–893.

Linderoth, B. and Håkanson, S., Retrogasserian glycerol rhizolysis in trigeminal neuralgia. In: H.H. Schmidek and W.H. Sweet (Eds.), Operative Neurosurgical Techniques, 3rd ed., Saunders, Philadelphia, 1995, pp. 1523–1536.

Lipton, S., Percutaneous cordotomy. In: P.D. Wall and R. Melzack (Eds.), Textbook of Pain, 2nd ed., Churchill Livingstone, Edinburgh, 1989, pp. 832–839.

Loeser, J.D., Tic douloureux and atypical face pain. In: P.D. Wall and R. Melzack (Eds.), Textbook of Pain, 3rd ed., Churchill Livingstone, Edinburgh, 1994, pp. 699–710.

Loeser, J.D., Sweet, W.H., Ten, J.W. Jr., Van Loveren, H. and Bonica, J.J., Neurosurgical operations involving peripheral nerves. In: J.J. Bonica (Ed.), The Management of Pain, 2nd ed., Lea & Febiger, Philadelphia, 1990, pp. 2044–2067.

Meyerson, B.A., Electric stimulation of the spinal cord and brain. In: J.J. Bonica (Ed.), The Management of Pain, 2nd ed., Lea & Febiger, Philadelphia, 1990, pp. 1862–1877.

Miles, J., Pituitary destruction. In: P.D. Wall and R. Melzack (Eds.), Textbook of Pain, 3rd ed., Churchill Livingstone, Edinburgh, 1994, pp. 1159–1170.

Nashold, J.R.B. and Nashold, B.S., Jr., Microsurgical DREZotomy in treatment of deafferentation pain. In: H.H. Schmidek and W.H. Sweet (Eds.), Operative Neurosurgical Techniques, 3rd ed., Saunders, Philadelplhia, 1995, pp. 1623–1636.

North, R.B., Spinal cord stimulation for chronic intractable pain. In: H.H. Schmidek and W.H. Sweet (Eds.), Operative Neurosurgical Techniques, 3rd ed., Saunders, Philadelphia, 1995, pp. 1403–1411.

North, R.B., Han, M., Zahurak, M. and Kidd, D.H., Radiofrequency lumbar facet denervation: analysis of prognostic factors, Pain, 57 (1994) 77–83.

Portenoy, R.K., Issues in the management of neuropathic pain. In: A.I. Basbaum and J.-M. Besson (Eds.), Towards a New Pharmacotherapy of Pain, Wiley & Sons, 1991, pp. 393–414.

Sweet, W.H., Treatment of trigeminal neuralgia by percutaneous rhizotomy. In: J.R. Youmans (Ed.), Neurological Surgery: A Comprehensive Reference Guide to the Diagnosis and Management of Neurosurgical Problems, 3rd ed., Saunders, Philadelphia, 1990, pp. 3888–3921.

Sweet, W.H. and Poletti, C.E., Operations in the brain stem and spinal canal, with an appendix on open cordotomy. In: P.D. Wall and R. Melzack (Eds.), Textbook of Pain, 3rd ed., Churchill Livingstone, Edinburgh, 1994, pp. 1113–1135.

Sweet, W.H. and Poletti, C.E., Complications of percutaneous decompression operations for facial pain. In: H.H. Schmidek and W.H. Sweet (Eds.), Operative Neurosurgical Techniques, 3rd ed., Saunders, Philadelphia, 1995, pp. 1543–1555.

Tasker, R.R., The problem of deafferentation pain in the management of the patient with cancer, J. Palliat. Care, 2 (1987) 8.

Tasker, R.R., Stereotactic surgery. In: P.D. Wall and R. Melzack (Eds.), Textbook of Pain, 3rd ed., Churchill Livingstone, Edinburgh, 1994a, pp. 1137–1157.

Tasker, R.R., The recurrence of pain after neurosurgical procedures, Quality of Life Research, Vol. 3, 1994b, Suppl. 1, pp. 543–549.

Tasker, R.R., Percutaneous cordotomy. In: H.H. Schmidek and W.H. Sweet (Eds.), Operative Neurosurgical Techniques, 3rd ed., Saunders, Philadelphia, 1995, pp. 1595–1611.

Tasker, R.R. and Dostrovsky, J.O., Deafferentation and central pain. In: P.D. Wall and R. Melzack (Eds.), Textbook of Pain, 2nd ed., Churchill Livingstone, Edinburgh, 1989, pp. 154–180.

Tasker, R.R. and Lougheed, W.M., Neurosurgical techniques of sympathetic interruption. In: M. Stanton-Hicks (Ed.), Pain and the Sympathetic Nervous System, Kluwer, Boston, 1990, pp. 165–190.

Taub, A., Robinson, F. and Taub, E., Dorsal root ganglionectomy for intractable monoradicular sciatica. In: H.H. Schmidek and W.H. Sweet (Eds.), Operative Neurosurgical Techniques, 3rd ed., Saunders, Philadelphia, 1995, pp. 1585–1593.

Willis, W.D., The pain system: The neural basis of nociceptive transmission. In: P.L. Gildenberg (Ed.), The Mammalian Nervous System, Pain and Headache, Vol. 8, Karger, Basel, 1985.

Wood, K.M., Peripheral nerve and root chemical lesions. In: P.D. Wall and R. Melzack (Eds.), Textbook of Pain, 2nd ed., Churchill Livingstone, Edinburgh, 1989, pp. 768–772.

White, J.C. and Sweet, W.H., Pain and the Neurosurgeon, Charles C. Thomas, Springfield, 1969.

Young, R.F. and Rinaldi, P.C., Brain Stimulation. In: P.D. Wall and R. Melzack (Eds.), Textbook of Pain, 3rd ed., Churchill Livingstone, Edinburgh, 1994, pp. 1225–1233.

Core Curriculum for Professional Education in Pain, edited by H.L. Fields, IASP Press, Seattle, © 1995.

13

Nerve Blocks

I. Know the anatomy of the following critical peripheral and central nervous system (CNS) regions as it relates to analgesic nerve blocks (Cousins and Bromage 1988; Hogan 1991; Abram and Boas 1992; Chambers 1993).

   A. Spine

   1. Bony vertebral column
   2. Spinal cord, meninges, nerve roots, dorsal root ganglion

   B. Peripheral nervous system

   1. Brachial, femoral, and sacral plexuses
   2. Cranial nerves
   3. Peripheral nerves of spinal origin: emphasis on nerves that are commonly involved in entrapment neuropathies, e.g., lateral femoral cutaneous, occipital, ulnar, median

   C. Autonomic nervous system

   1. Sympathetic efferent system

      a. Cells or origin in spinal cord
      b. Rami communicantes
      c. Sympathetic chain
      d. Postganglionics

   2. Visceral (sympathetic) afferent system

      a. Innervation of visceral structures
      b. Sympathetic chain afferents from somatic structures

II. Be familiar with the general principles of the pharmacology of drugs used for nerve blocks.

   A. Local anesthetics (Covino 1988; Charlton 1993)

   1. Neural blocking mechanisms
   2. Be aware of the systemic effects

      a. CNS toxic effects
      b. Nonconvulsant effects (e.g., analgesia)
      c. Cardiotoxic effects

3. Pharmacokinetics (Tucker and Mather 1988)

    a. Peripheral nerve block
    b. Subarachnoid block
    c. Epidural block

B. Know the pharmacology of opiates as they relate to regional analgesia (Cousins and Mather 1984; Martin 1984; Mather and Phillips 1986; Cousins et al. 1988a; Dickinson 1991; McQuay 1991).

1. Receptor types and function
2. Spinal and brain effects
3. Pharmacokinetics of spinal intrathecal and epidural application

C. Know the commonly used neurolytic agents (Myers and Katz 1988).

1. Alcohol, phenol
2. Pathological (neurotoxic) effects

    a. Blood vessels
    b. Spinal cord

3. Know the complications of neurolytic therapy (Swerdlow 1980).

    a. Denervation dysesthesia
    b. Peripheral neuralgia

D. Know about the use of locally injected corticosteroids (Rowlingson 1994).

1. Effect on nerve roots, peripheral nerves
2. Systemic effects
3. Pharmacokinetics of soluble, "depo" preparations

III. Know how nerve blocks are used for diagnostic purposes and pain control (Abram and Haddox 1992; Hogan and Abram, in press). All practitioners should understand the clinical indications, risks, and complications associated with the use of nerve blocks. All practitioners, including those outside of the field of anesthesiology, should be aware of the treatment of problems that may arise during the performance of these procedures.

A. Myofascial trigger point injection

B. Common peripheral blocks (Abram and Haddox 1992)

1. Occipital
2. Lateral femoral cutaneous
3. Intercostal

C. Sympathetic blocks (Abram and Boas 1992; Abram and Haddox 1992)

1. Lumbar sympathetic
2. Stellate ganglion

D. Epidural steroid injections (Benzon 1966; Myers and Katz 1988)

E. Celiac plexus block and hypogastric plexus block (Plancarte et al. 1993)

F. Intraspinal opiates

    1. Techniques of catheter placement: intrathecal, epidural
    2. Administration techniques

        a. Bolus
        b. External infusion
        c. Subcutaneous post
        d. Implantable infusion pump

G. Intrathecal and epidural neurolytic blocks (Cousins et al. 1988b)

H. Phenol motor point block (Halpern and Meelhuysen 1966)

IV. Know how to recognize and treat the side effects and complications of nerve blocks (Abram and Hogan 1992; Murphy and O'Keefe 1992).

A. Spinal and epidural blocks

B. Paravertabral somatic and sympathetic blocks

C. Peripheral nerve blocks

D. Muscle, joint, and bursa injections

E. Continuous infusion therapy

REFERENCES

Abram, S.E. and Boas, R.A., Sympathetic and visceral nerve blocks. In: J.L. Benumot (Ed.), Procedures in Anesthesia and Intensive Care, J.B. Lippincott, Philadelphia, 1992, pp. 787–806.

Abram, S.E. and Hogan, Q.H., Complications of peripheral nerve blocks. In: L. Saidman and J. Benumof (Eds.), Anesthesia and Perioperative Complications, C.V. Mosby, St. Louis, 1992, pp. 52–76.

Abram, S.E. and Haddox, J.D., Chronic pain management. In: P.G. Barash, B.F. Cullen and R.K. Stoelting (Eds.), Clinical Anesthesia, 2nd ed., J.B. Lippincott, Philadelphia, 1992, pp. 1579–1607.

Benzon, H.T., Epidural steroid injections for low back pain and lumbosacral radiculopathy, Pain, 24 (1966) 277.

Carpenter, R.L. and Mackey, D.C., Local anesthetics. In: P.G. Barash, B.F. Cullen. and R.K. Stoelting (Eds.), Clinical Anesthesia, J.B. Lippincott, Philadelphia, 1989, pp. 371–403.

Chambers, W.A., Anatomy of the spine. In: J.A.W. Wildsmith and E.N. Armitage (Eds.), Principles and Practice of Regional Anesthesia, 2nd ed., Churchill Livingtone, Edinburgh, 1993, pp. 77–85.

Charlton, J.E., The management of regional anesthesia. In: J.A.W. Wildsmith and E.N. Armitage (Eds.), Principles and Practice of Regional Anesthesia, 2nd ed., Churchill Livingtone, Edinburgh, 1993, pp. 47–75.

Cousins, M.J. and Bromage, P.R., Epidural neural blockade. In: M.J. Cousins and P.O. Bridenbaugh (Eds.), Neural Blockade, 2nd ed., J.B. Lippincott, Philadelphia, 1988, pp. 253–360.

Cousins, M.J. and Mather, L.E., Intrathecal and epidural administration of opioids, Anesthesiology, 61 (1984) 276.

Cousins, M.J., Cherry, D.A. and Gourlay, G.K., Acute and chronic pain: use of spinal opioids. In: M.J. Cousins and P.O. Bridenbaugh (Eds.), Neural Blockade in Clinical Anesthesia and Management of Pain, 2nd ed., J.B. Lippincott, Philadelphia, 1988, pp. 955–1029.

Cousins, M.J., Dwyer, B. and Gibb, D., Chronic pain and neurolytic blockade. In: M.J. Cousins and P.O. Bridenbaugh (Eds.), Neural Blockade in Clinical Anesthesia and Management of Pain, 2nd ed., J.B. Lippincott, Philadelphia, 1988, pp. 1053–1084.

Covino, B.C., Clinical pharmacology of local anesthetic agents. In: M.J. Cousins and P.O. Bridenbaugh (Eds.), Neural Blockade, 2nd ed., J.B. Lippincott, Philadelphia, 1988, pp. 111–144.

Dickinson, A.H., Mechanism of the analgesic actions of opiates and opioids, Br. Med. Bull., 47 (1991) 690–702.

Halpern, D. and Meelhuysen, F.E., Phenol motor point block in the management of muscular hypertonia, Arch. Phys. Med. Rehab., 47 (1966) 659–664.

Hogan, Q.H. and Abram, S.E., The diagnostic use of nerve blocks, In: P.O. Bridenbaugh and M.J. Cousins (Eds.), Neural Blockade, 3rd ed., J.B. Lippincott, Philadelphia, in press.

Hogan, Q.H., Lumbar epidural anatomy, Anesthesiology, 75 (1991) 767–775.

Martin, W.R., Pharmacology of opioids, Pharmacol Rev., 35, (1984) 283–323.

Mather, L.E. and Phillips, G.D., Opioids and adjuvants: principles of use. In: M.J. Cousins and G.D. Phillips (Eds.), Acute Pain Management, Churchill Livingstone, New York, 1986, pp. 77–103.

McQuay, H.J., Opioid clinical pharmacology and routes of administration, Br. Med. Bull., 47 (1991) 703–717.

Murphy, T.M. and O'Keefe, D., Complications of spinal, epidural, and caudal anesthesia. In: J.L. Benumof and L.J. Saidman (Eds.), Anesthesia and Perioperative Complications, Mosby–Year Book, Chicago, 1992, pp. 38–51.

Myers, R.R. and Katz, J., Neuropathology of neurolytic and semidestructive agents. In: M.J. Cousins and P.O. Bridenbaugh (Eds.), Neural Blockade, 2nd ed., J.B. Lippincott, Philadelphia, 1988, pp. 1031–1052.

Plancarte, R., Amescua, C., Patt, R.B. and Aldrete, J.A., Superior hypogastric plexus block for pelvic cancer pain, Anesthesiology, 73 (1993) 236–239.

Rowlingson, J.C., Epidural Steroids, APS Journal, 3 (1994) 20–32.

Scott, D.B., Techniques of Regional Anaesthesia, Appleton and Lange, Norwalk, 1989.

Swerdlow, M., Complications of neurolytic neural blockade, In: P.O. Bridenbaugh and M.J. Cousins (Eds.), Neural Blockade, 1st ed., J.B. Lippincott, Philadelphia, 1980, pp. 543–556.

Travell, J.A. and Simons, D.G., Myofascial Pain and Dysfunction: The Trigger Point Manual, Vol. 1, Williams & Wilkins, Baltimore, 1983.

Tucker, J.A. and Mather, L.E., Properties, absorption and distribution of local anesthetic agents. In: M.J. Cousins and P.O. Bridenbaugh (Eds.), Neural Blockade, 2nd ed., J.B. Lippincott, Philadelphia, 1988, pp. 47–110.

Core Curriculum for Professional Education in Pain, edited by H.L. Fields, IASP Press, Seattle, © 1995.

14

Psychiatric Evaluation and Treatment

I. Be able to make a diagnosis of major depression or dysthymic disorder, and to distinguish these forms of mental disorder from the depressive symptoms that often accompany chronic pain. The diagnosis must be based on a clinical examination, including a detailed mental state evaluation, and not solely on a questionnaire (Pilowsky and Bassett 1982).

II. Know the indications for the use of antidepressants. Be able to recommend appropriate doses and times of administration for patients who have affective disorders. Be able to use antidepressants for pain patients: e.g., amitriptyline, and know the evidence for their analgesic effect in the absence of depression (Goodkin and Gullion 1989; Ward 1986).

III. Be aware of the different forms of psychotherapy for depression including supportive, cognitive, behavioral, marital and family, interpretative and group (Flor et al. 1987; Turner 1988; Pilowsky and Barrow 1990; Flor et al. 1992).

IV. Be able to discriminate anxiety conditions in which treatment to relieve anxiety is of prime importance. Understand the application of the different forms of psychotherapy for anxiety disorders, for example, supportive, cognitive, behavioral, marital and family, interpretative and group (Turk and Rudy 1986; Flor et al. 1987; Keefe et al. 1992). Note that chronic pain patients reporting greater anxiety have a tendency to overpredict new pain events (McCracken et al. 1993) and that high anxiety may disrupt the use of self-control strategies in coping with pain (McCracken and Gross 1993; Biedermann and Schefft 1994).

V. Be aware that anger is an emotion that is frequently seen in chronic pain patients (Wade et al. 1990; Kerns et al. 1994) and that anger intensity relates to perceived pain interference (Kerns et al. 1994). Anger may be a specific affective component of pain along with fear and sadness (Fernandez and Milburn 1994) and may be an important concomitant of the depression in chronic pain (Wade et al. 1990). In psychiatric patients "anger attacks" may be possible variants of panic and major depression (Fava et al. 1990). The presence of anger in a chronic pain patient should alert the pain physician to a syndrome that may be treatable by psychopharmacology.

VI. Understand the controversy over opiate medication and detoxification for the chronic pain patient (Chabal et al. 1992; Fishbain et al. 1992a; Sees and Clark 1992; Jamison et al. 1994) and be aware of the protocols for opiate and sedative detoxification (Fishbain et al. 1992b; Fishbain et al. 1993).

VII. Understand the application of supportive psychotherapy, reassurance and limited rexamination, sympathetic discussion and redirection of interest, for patients with somatoform disorders and hypochondriasis. Appreciate that supportive relationships can be effective for hypochondriacal patients. Understand the application of the other techniques recommended for patients with somatization disorder and hypochondriasis, including supportive, cognitive, behavioral, marital and family therapy (Adler 1981; Lazare 1981; Ford and Folk 1985; Ford 1986; Lipowski 1988; Orenstein 1989; Tunks and Merskey 1990; Merskey 1994).

VIII. Know the value of interviewing a spouse or other relatives and evaluating information about the case obtained from a relative. Understand that discussions leading up to an appreciation by all parties of the implications of pain, and other social or interpersonal problems are often of value in management (Feuerstein et al. 1985; Sternbach 1986; Flor et al. 1987; Flor et al. 1992).

IX. Understand the importance of coping strategies for the control of pain and the current status of this area of pain treatment research (Jensen et al. 1991). Understand that coping strategies may differ between individuals and may be affected by age and gender (Elton et al. 1994).

X. A large percentage of chronic pain patients complain of sleep disturbance. Sleep laboratory analyses show that they sleep less than do insomniacs and demonstrate nocturnal myoclonus and alpha intrusions (Atkinson et al. 1988a, 1988b). Patients with high pain intensities report significantly less sleep (Atkinson et al. 1988a).These sleep disturbances are usually treated with tricyclic antidepressants or hypnotics (Fishbain et al. 1992a).

XI. Understand that in seeking medical care, chronic pain patients may have treatment goals that differ widely from those of the treating professional (Hazard et al. 1993); a patient's satisfaction with care will be determined by whether his or her goals for treatment are met (Hazard et al. 1993).

XII. Know the value of encouragement and of assisting the person to identify major problems in his or her life or circumstances. Be able to recognize when these problems require specialist attention (Feuerstein et al.1985; Howard 1985).

XIII. Know the value of evaluation of the patient's past work level and educational attainment and be able to refer patients for appropriate psychological testing for both intellectual capacity and vocational preference. Be able to identify patients for whom vocational guidance, further education, and retraining may lead to rehabilitation (Weinstein 1978; Feuerstein et al. 1985; Sternbach 1986).

XIV. Be able to advise on the effects of chronic pain upon the personality, to provide insight and support for the patient, to interpret the situation to the family and other relatives and interested persons, and to advise on cognitive treatments. Be able to introduce suitable cognitive and behavioral measures or recognize when it is appropriate to refer for the patient for special evaluation and therapy (Atkinson et al. 1988a; Flor et al. 1987; Sternbach 1986).

XV. Be able to advise on adaptation to chronic pain in the light of the above guidelines (Edwards 1982; Howard 1985).

REFERENCES

Adler, G., The physician and the hypochondriacal patient, N. Engl. J. Med., 304 (1981) 1394–1396.

Atkinson, J.H., Slater, M.A., Grant, I., Patterson, T.L. and Garfin, S.R., Depressed mood in chronic low back pain: Relationship with stressful life events, Pain, 35 (1988a) 47–55.

Atkinson, J.H., Ancoli-Israel, S., Slater, M.A., Garfin, S.R. and Gillin, J.C., Subjective sleep disturbance in chronic back pain, Clin. J. Pain, 4 (1988b) 225–232.

Biedermann J.J. and Schefft, B.K., Behavioral, physiological, and self-evaluative effects of anxiety on the self-control of pain, Behav. Modif. 18, (1994) 89–105.

Chabal, C., Jacobson, L., Chaney, E.F. and Mariano, A.J., Narcotics for chronic pain, Yes or No? A useless dichotomy, APS Journal, 1 (1992) 376–381.

Edwards, L.D., Psychiatric, psychological and some physiological influences on the response to pain treatment: a review, Methods Find. Exp. Clin. Pharmacol., 4 (1982) 511–520.

Elton, N.H., Magdi, M.H., Treasure, J. and Treasure, H., Coping with chronic pain: some patients suffer more, Brit. J. Psychiat., 165 (1994) 802–807.

Fava, M., Anderson, F.M., Fava, H., Anderson, K. and Rosenbaum, J.F., "Anger attacks": Possible variants of panic and major depressive disorders, Am. J. Psychiat., 147 (1990) 867–870.

Fernandez, E. and Milburn, T.W., Sensory and affective predictors of overall pain and emotions associated with affective pain, Clin. J. Pain, 10 (1994) 3–9.

Feuerstein, M., Sult, S. and Houle, M., Environmental stressors and chronic low back pain: life events, family and work environment, Pain, 22 (1985) 295–307.

Fishbain, D.A., Rosomoff, H.L. and Rosomofff, R.S., Drug abuse, dependence, and addiction in chronic pain patients, Clin. J. Pain, 8 (1992a) 77–85.

Fishbain, D. A., Rosomoff, H. L. and Rosomoff, R. S., Detoxification of nonopiate drugs in the chronic pain setting and Clonidine opiate detoxification, Clin. J. Pain, 8 (1992b) 191–203.

Fishbain, D.A., Rosomoff, H.L., Cutler, R. and Rosomoff, R.S., Opiate detoxification protocols, Ann. Clin. Psych., 5 (1993) 53–65.

Flor, H., Turk, D.C. and Rudy, T.E., Pain and families II. Assessment and treatment, Pain, 30 (1987) 29–45.

Flor, H., Fydrich, T. and Turk, D.C., Efficacy of multi-disciplinary pain treatment centers: a meta-analytic review, Pain, 49 (1992) 221–230.

Ford, C.V., The somatizing disorders: Psychosomatics, 27 (1986) 327–337.

Ford, C.V. and Folk, D.G., Conversion disorders: an overview, Psychosomatics, 26 (1985) 371–381.

Goodkin, K. and Gullion, C.M., Antidepressants for the relief of chronic pain: do they work? Ann. Behav. Med., 11 (1989) 83–101.

Hazard, R.G., Haugh, L.D., Green, P.A. and Jones, P.L., Chronic low back pain: the relationship between patient satisfaction and pain, impairment, and disability outcomes, Spine, 19 (1993) 881–887

Howard, L.R., The stress and strain of pain, Stress Med., 1 (1985) 41–46.

Jamison, R.N., Anderson, K.O., Peeters-Asdourian, C. and Ferrante, F.M., Survey of opiod use in chronic nonmalignant pain patients, Reg. Anesth., 19 (1994) 225–230.

Jensen, M.P., Turner, J.A., Romano, J.M. and Karoly, P., Coping with chronic pain: a critical review of the literature, Pain, 47 (1991) 249–283.

Keefe, F.J., Dunsmore, J. and Burnett, R., Behavioral and cognitive-behavioral approaches to chronic pain: recent advances and future directions, J. Consult. Clin. Psychol., 60 (1992) 528–536

Kerns, R.D., Rosenberg, R. and Jacon, M.C., Anger expression and chronic pain, J. Behav. Med., 17 (1994) 57–62.

Lazare, A., Conversion symptoms, N. Engl. J. Med., 305 (1981) 745–748.

Lipowski, Z.J., Somatization: the concept and first clinical application, Am. J. Psychiatry, 145 (1988) 1358–1368.

McCracken, L.M. and Gross, R.T., Does anxiety affect coping with chronic pain? Clin. J. Pain, 9 (1993) 253–259.

McCracken, L.M., Gross, R.T., Sorg, P.J. and Edmands, T.A., Prediction of pain in patients with chronic low back pain: effects of inaccurate prediction and pain-related anxiety, Behav. Res. Ther., 31 (1993) 647–652.

Merskey, H., Pain and psychological medicine. In: P.D. Wall and R. Melzack (Eds.), Textbook of Pain, 3rd ed., Churchill Livingston, Edinburgh, 1994, pp. 903–920.

Orenstein, H., Briquet's syndrome in association with depression and panic: a reconceptualization of Briquet's syndrome, Am. J. Psychiatry, 146 (1989) 334–338.

Pilowsky, I. and Bassett, D.L., Pain and depression, Brit. J. Psychiatry, 141 (1982) 30–36.

Pilowsky, I. and Barrow, C.G., A controlled study of psychotherapy and amitriptyline used individually and in combination in the treatment of chronic intractable (psychogenic) pain, Pain, 40 (1990) 3–19.

Sees, K.L. and Clark, H.W., Opioid use in the treatment of chronic pain: assessment of addiction, J. Pain Symptom Manage., 8 (1992) 257–264.

Sternbach, R.A. (Ed.), The Psychology of Pain, 2nd ed., Raven Press, New York, 1986.

Tunks, E. and Merskey, H., Psychotherapy of pain. In: J.J. Bonica (Ed.), The Management of Pain, 2nd ed., Lea & Febiger, Philadelphia, 1990.

Turk, D.C. and Rudy, T.E., Assessment of cognitive factors in chronic pain: a worthwhile enterprise? J. Consult Clin. Psychol., 54 (1986) 760–768.

Turner, J.A., Comparison of operant behavioral and cognitive behavioral group treatment for chonic low back pain, J. Consult. Clin. Psychol., 56 (1988) 261–266.

Wade, J.B., Price, D.D., Hamer, R.M. and Schwartz, S.M., An emotional component analysis of chronic pain, Pain, 40 (1990) 303–310.

Ward, N.G., Tricyclic antidepressants for chronic low back pain: mechanism of action and predictors of response, Spine, 11 (1986) 661–665.

Weinstein, M.R., The concept of the disability process, Psychosomatics, 19 (1978) 94–97.

Core Curriculum for Professional Education in Pain, edited by H.L. Fields, IASP Press, Seattle, © 1995.

15

Psychological Treatments (Behavioral Interventions)

I. For the following intervention strategies, understand the theoretical rationale, assessment procedures, indications, specific details of the treatment approach, and efficacy (Turner and Chapman 1982a,b; Flor et al. 1992; Keefe et al. 1992; Turk and Melzack 1992).

  A. Know about relaxation strategies: progressive muscle relaxation, autogenic training, guided imagery, cue-controlling, and other strategies (Turner and Chapman 1982a; Jessup and Gallegos 1994).

  B. Know the cognitive behavioral treatments of pain: stress innoculation training, cognitive-therapy, and rational emotive therapy (Turner and Chapman 1982b; Turk et al. 1983; Turk and Meichenbaum 1994).

  C. Understand operant therapy: contingency management for pain and well behavior, exercise management, medication management, etc. (Fordyce 1976; Keefe and Lefebvre 1994).

  D. Be familiar with biofeedback, using: electromyographic (EMG), temperature, blood pressure, electroencephalographic (EEG) feedback, etc. (Turk and Flor 1984; Flor and Birbaumer 1993; Jessup and Gallegos 1994).

  E. Be familiar with hypnoanalgesia and other hypnotic effects (Hilgard 1986; Spanos 1986; Spanos et al. 1994).

  F. Be familiar with preparation strategies for postoperative pain (Peterson and Mori 1988).

  G. Understand social skills training; focus on preparation and rehabilitation of the patient for vocational, family, and daily activities (Fordyce et al. 1985; Fedoravicius and Klein 1986).

  H. Be familiar with modelling therapies and observational learning (Craig 1986; Elkins and Roberts 1985).

  I. Be aware of group therapy and how to assess patients for likely efficacy of approaches (Gamsa et al. 1985; Turner 1988).

  J. Be familiar with behavioral strategies for enhancing adherence to therapeutic regimes (Meichenbaum and Turk 1987; Holroyd et al. 1988).

  K. Be familiar with family system management (Flor et al. 1987; Roy 1986).

  L. Be familiar with relapse prevention (Linton et al. 1989; Turk and Rudy 1991; McGrath and Manion, in press).

II. Be familiar with how the various separate approaches can be integrated (Turk et al. 1983; Philips 1988; Flor and Birbaumer 1991).

III. Recognize common process factors in behavioral interventions: rapport, communication strategies, support, persussion, trust, suggestion, etc. (Turk and Holzman 1986).

IV. Know the role of clinical decision-making: selecting a treatment modality for the patient and matching interventions to patients (Cameron and Shepel 1986; Turk and Rudy 1986; Flor and Birbaumer 1991).

V. Recognize the application of various behavioral strategies to specific pain syndromes: dental pain, low back pain, burn pain, postoperative pain, etc. (Burrows et al. 1987; McGrath and Unruh 1987; Wall and Melzack 1994).

VI. Recognize behavioral components and importance of social context of all biological interventions (motivational factors, relationship factors, suggestion, trust, adherence) (Kendall 1983; Bond 1984; Turk and Rudy 1991).

REFERENCES

Bond, M.R., Pain: Its Nature, Analysis and Treatment, 2nd ed., Churchill Livingstone, Edinburgh, 1984.

Burrows, G.D., Elton, D. and Stanley, G.V. (Eds.), Handbook of Chronic Pain Management, Elsevier Science Publishers, Amsterdam, 1987.

Cameron, R. and Shepel, L.F., The process of psychological consultation in pain management. In: A.D. Holzman and D.C. Turk (Eds.), Pain Management: A Handbook of Psychological Treatment Approaches, Guilford Press, New York, 1986, 240–256.

Craig, K.D., Social modeling influences: pain in context, In: R.A. Sternbach (Ed.), The Psychology of Pain, 2nd ed., Raven Press, New York, 1986, pp. 67–96.

Elkins, P.D. and Roberts, M.C., Reducing medical fears in a general population of children: a comparison of three audiovisual modeling procedures, J. Pediatr. Psychol., 10 (1985) 65–75.

Fedoravicius, A.S. and Klein, B.J., Social skills training in an outpatient medical setting. In: A.D. Holzman and D.C. Turk (Eds.), Pain Management: A Handbook of Psychological Treatment Approaches, Oxford, New York, 1986, pp. 86–99.

Flor, H. and Birbaumer, N., Comprehensive assessment and treatment of chronic back-pain patients without physical disabilities. In: M.R. Bond, J.E. Charlton and C.J. Woolf (Eds.), Proceedings of the VIth World Congress on Pain, Pain Research and Clinical Management, Vol. 4., Elsevier, Amsterdam, 1991, pp. 229–234.

Flor, H. and Birbaumer, N., Comparison of EMG-biofeedback, cognitive behavior therapy, and conservative medical treatment for chronic musculoskeletal pain, J. Consult. Clin. Psychol., 61 (1993) 653–658.

Flor, H., Fydrich, T. and Turk, D.C., Efficacy of multi-disciplinary pain treatment centers: a meta-analytic review, Pain, 49 (1992) 221–230.

Flor, H., Turk, D.C. and Rudy, T.E., Pain and families, II. Assessment and treatment, Pain, 30 (1987) 251–260.

Fordyce, W.E., Behavioral Methods for Chronic Pain and Illness, C.V. Mosby, St. Louis, 1976.

Fordyce, W.E., Roberts, A.H. and Sternbach, R.A., The behavioral management of chronic pain: a response to critics, Pain, 22 (1985) 113–126.

Gamsa, A., Braha, R.E.D. and Catchlove, R.F.H., The use of structured group therapy sessions in the treatment of chronic pain patients, Pain, 22 (1985) 91–96.

Hilgard, E.R., Hypnosis and pain. In: R.A. Sternbach (Ed.), The Psychology of Pain, 2nd ed., Raven Press, New York, 1986.

Holroyd, K.A., Holm, J.E., Hursey, K.G., Penzien, D.B., Cordingley, G.E., Theofanus, A.G., Richardson, S.C. and Tobin, D.L., Recurrent vascular headache: home-based behavioral treatment versus abortive pharmacological treatment, J. Consult. Clin. Psychol., 56 (1988) 218–223.

Jessup, B.A. and Gallegos, X., Relaxation and biofeedback. In: P.D. Wall and R. Melzack (Eds.), Textbook of Pain, 3rd ed., Churchil Livingstone, Edinburgh, 1994, pp. 1321–1336.

Keefe, F.J. and Lefebvre, J.C., Behaviour therapy. In: P.D. Wall and R. Melzack (Eds.), Textbook of Pain, 3rd ed., Churchill Livingstone, Edinburgh, 1994, pp. 1367–1380.

Keefe, F.J., Dunsmore, J. and Burnett, R., Behavioral and cognitive-behavioral approaches to chronic pain: recent advances and future directions, J. Consult. Clin. Psychol., 60 (1992) 528–536.

Kendall, P.C., Stressful medical procedures: cognitive-behavioral strategies for stress management and prevention. In: D.H. Meichenbaum and M.E. Jaremko (Eds.), Stress Reduction and Prevention, Plenum, New York, 1983, pp. 159–190.

Linton, S.J., Bradley, L.A., Jensen, E., Spangfort, E. and Sundell, L., The secondary prevention of low back pain: a controlled study with follow-up, Pain, 36 (1989) 197–208.

McGrath, P.J. and Manion, I.G., Prevention of pain problems. In: K.D. Craig and S.M. Weiss (Eds.), Health Enhancement, Disease Prevention and Early Intervention: Biobehavioral Perspectives, Springer, New York, 1990.

McGrath, P.J. and Unruh, A.M., Pain in Children and Adolescents, Elsevier Science Publishers, Amsterdam, 1987.

Meichenbaum, D. and Turk, D.C., Facilitating treatment adherence, Plenum, New York, 1987.

Peterson, L.J. and Mori, L., Preparation for hospitalization. In: D.K. Routh (Ed.), Handbook of Pediatric Psychology, Guilford Press, New York, 1988.

Philips, H.C., The Psychological Management of Chronic Pain: A Treatment Manual, Springer Publishing Company, New York, 1988.

Roy, R., A problem-centered family systems approach in treating chronic pain. In: A.D. Holzman and D.C. Turk (Eds.), Pain Management: A Handbook of Psychological Treatment Approaches, Oxford, New York, pp. 113–130.

Spanos, N.P., Hypnotic behavior: a social-psychological interpretation of amnesia, analgesia and "trance-logic." Behavior and Brain Science, 9 (1986) 449–502.

Spanos, N.P., Carmanico, S.J. and Ellis, J.A., Hypnotic analgesia. In: P.D. Wall and R. Melzack (Eds.), Textbook of Pain, 3rd ed., Churchill Livingstone, Edinburgh, 1994, pp. 1349–1366.

Turk, D.C. and Flor, H., Etiological theories and treatments for chronic back pain. II. Psychological models and interventions, Pain, 19 (1984) 209–233.

Turk, D.C. and Holzman, A.D., Commonalities among psychological approaches in the treatment of chronic pain: specifying the meta-constructs. In: A.D. Holzman and D.C. Turk (Eds.), Pain Management: A Handbook of Psychological Treatment Approaches, Oxford, New York, 1986, pp. 257–267.

Turk, D.C. and Meichenbaum, D., A cognitive-behavioral approach to pain management. In: P.D. Wall and R. Melzack (Eds.), Textbook of Pain, 3rd ed., Churchill Livingstone, Edinburgh, 1994, pp. 1337–1348.

Turk, D.C., Meichenbaum, D.H. and Genest, M., Pain and Behavioral Medicine: A Cognitive-behavioral Perspective, Guilford Press, New York, 1983.

Turk, D.C. and Melzack, R., The measurement of pain and the assessment of people experiencing pain. In: D.C. Turk and R. Melzack (Eds.), Handbook of Pain Assessment, Guilford Press, New York, 1992, pp. 3–12.

Turk, D.C. and Rudy, T.E., Assessment of cognitive factors in chronic pain: a worthwhile enterprise? J. Consult. Clin. Psychol., 54 (1986) 760–768.

Turk, D.C. and Rudy, T.E., Neglected topics in the treatment of chronic pain patients: relapse, noncompliance and adherence enhancement, Pain, 44 (1991) 5–28.

Turner, J.A., Comparison of operant behavioral and cognitive behavioral group treatment for chronic low back pain, J. Consult. Clin. Psychol., 56 (1988) 261–266.

Turner, J.A. and Chapman, C.R., Psychological interventions for chronic pain: a critical review, I. Relaxation training and biofeedback, Pain, 12, (1982a) 1–21.

Turner, J.A. and Chapman, C.R., Psychological interventions for chronic pain: a critical review, II. Operant conditioning, hypnosis and cognitive behavior therapy, Pain, 12 (1982b) 23–46.

Wall, P.D. and Melzack, R. (Eds.), Textbook of Pain, 3rd ed., Churchill Livingstone, Edinburgh, 1994.

Core Curriculum for Professional Education in Pain, edited by H.L. Fields, IASP Press, Seattle, © 1995.

16

Multidisciplinary Pain Management

I. Understand the purpose of a multidisciplinary pain clinic (MPC), the common reasons for patient referrals, and the range of patient problems frequently encountered (Loeser and Egan 1989; Loeser et al. 1990; Schwartz 1991).

II. Know the range of services that multidisciplinary pain clinics provide (Loeser and Egan 1989; Loeser et al. 1990; Cohen and Campbell, in press).

III. Define multidisciplinary as it relates to pain management. Distinguish MPCs from other forms of pain clinics (Loeser and Egan 1989).

IV. Understand the effects of chronicity upon patients with pain (Fordyce 1976; Loeser et al. 1990).

V. Know why a multidisciplinary approach is of particular value for patients with chronic pain. Be familiar with published studies of outcome of patients treated by this approach. Know how outcomes studies are conducted (Fordyce 1976; Flor et al. 1992; Deyo 1993; Turk et al. 1993).

VI. List the types of qualification and functions of health care professionals that would participate in an ideal MPC. Know what each contributes (Ghia 1992; Loeser and Egan 1989; Pilowski 1976).

VII. Know the types of problems that require an inpatient as opposed to an outpatient pain management program (Loeser and Egan 1989; Schwartz 1991).

VIII. Be familiar with the evaluation process, the clinical issues that are addressed, the staff that are involved, and the strategies for developing a treatment plan (Loeser and Egan 1989; Loeser et al. 1990).

IX. Know the practical aspects of administering an MPC (Pilowski 1976; Loeser and Egan 1989; Campbell and Cohen, in press).

   A. Personnel

   B. Facilities

   C. Policies and practices

   D. Financial

X. Understand the interface of an MPC with the larger medical community. Know how MPCs establish continuity of care utilizing community resources. Know how an MPC can use consultants in evaluation and treatment of complex problems (Loeser and Egan 1989; Deyo 1993; Turk et al. 1993).

XI. Be familiar with the costs of patient evaluation and treatment for common problems that are encountered in funding pain clinics in your health care system. Be aware of how these costs compare with those for alternative treatment strategies (Pilowski 1976; Ghia 1992; Turk et al. 1993; Campbell and Cohen, in press).

REFERENCES

Cohen, M.J. and Campbell, J.N. (Eds.), Pain Treatment Centers at a Crossroads, IASP Press, Seattle, in press.

Deyo, R.A., Practice variations, treatment fads, rising disability, Spine, 18 (1993) 2153–2162.

Flor, H., Fydrich, T. and Turk, D.C., Efficacy of multidisciplinary pain treatment centers: a meta-analytic review, Pain, 49 (1992) 221–230.

Fordyce, W.E., Behavioral Methods for Chronic Pain and Illness, Mosby–Year Book, St. Louis, 1976.

Ghia, J.N., Development and organization of pain centers. In: P.P. Raj (Ed.), Practical Management of Pain, 2nd ed., Mosby, St. Louis, 1992, pp. 16–39.

Loeser, J.D. and Egan, K.J., Managing the Chronic Pain Patient: Theory and Practice at the University of Washington Multidisciplinary Pain Center, Raven Press, New York, 1989.

Loeser, J.D., Seres, J. and Newman, R.I., Jr., Interdisciplinary multimodal management of chronic pain. In: J.J. Bonica (Ed.), The Management of Pain, 2nd ed., Lea and Febiger, Philadelphia, 1990, pp. 2107–2120.

Pilowski, I., The psychiatrist and the pain clinic, Am. J. Psychiatry, 133 (1976) 752–756.

Schwartz, D.P., Appropriate referral to inpatient vs. outpatient pain management programs: a clinician's guide, Pain Digest, 1 (1991) 2–6.

Turk, D., Rudy, T.E. and Sorkin, B.A., Neglected topics in chronic pain treatment outcome studies: determination of success, Pain, 53 (1993) 3–16.

Core Curriculum for Professional Education in Pain, edited by H.L. Fields, IASP Press, Seattle, © 1995.

17

Taxonomy of Pain Syndromes

I.   Be familiar with the IASP classification of chronic pain syndromes, the principles upon which it is based, and the application to cases which are most commonly seen.

II. Be able to allocate the majority of patients to a specific diagnostic code or codes within the system.

III. Understand the applications of the definitions of pain terms.

REFERENCE

Merskey, H. and Bogduk, N. (Eds.), Classification of Chronic Pain: Descriptions of Chronic Pain Syndromes and Definitions of Pain Terms, 2nd ed., IASP Press, Seattle, 1994.

Core Curriculum for Professional Education in Pain, edited by H.L. Fields, IASP Press, Seattle, © 1995.

18

Low Back Pain

I. Know and understand the numerous diagnostic labels appended to the syndrome of low back pain, for example, lumbosacral sprain, lumbar discogenic syndromes, spondylolysis and listhesis, facet syndrome, lumbar spondylosis, spinal stenosis, unstable low back, low back disorders, failed back syndrome, and tropism. Recognize the lack of specificity of diagnosis for most patients with low back pain. Know the risk factors for significant underlying disease in patients with low back pain (Cailliet 1988; Borenstein and Wiesel 1989; Loeser 1990, 1991; Frymoyer 1993).

II. Know the functional anatomy of the lumbosacral spine (Cailliet 1988; Borenstein and Wiesel 1989; Frymoyer 1993; Bigos 1994).

   A. Know the components of a functional unit: vertebrae, zygapophyseal (facet) joints, intervertebral disc, ligaments, muscles, and posterior neural canal. Know the relationship of the nerve roots and their dural sheaths to this unit.

   B. Know the neuromuscular function of the spine. Understand the motion of the functional unit and its role in the "lumbar pelvic rhythm." Be aware of symmetric and asymmetric motion (Marras et al. 1993a).

   C. Know the nociceptor sites of the functional unit.

   D. Know how to examine these structures using a meaningful history and a physical examination.

   E. Be familiar with x-ray, magnetic resonance imaging (MRI), and computerized tomography findings in relation to the history and examination. Know the association between age and imaging findings and the poor correlation of pain complaints with imaging studies.

III. Know the common pathological changes in the lumbosacral spine area that are thought to produce pain, including (Cailliet 1988; Loeser 1990; Nachemson 1992):

   A. Mechanical and chemical consequences of disc degeneration, protrusion, annular tear

   B. Facet degenerative arthritis

   C. Foraminal and spinal stenosis

   D. Segmental scoliosis

   E. Lysis and lysthesis

IV.   Know the common causes of acute low back pain, recurrent low back pain, and chronic low back pain. Know their epidemiology and natural history (Cailliet 1988; Frymoyer and Cats-Baril 1991; Marras 1993; Back Pain 1994; Bigos 1994).

V.   Be aware of the physiological basis for the standard modalities for treating acute, recurrent, and chronic low back pain, including (Bartz 1984; Nachemson 1992; Frymoyer 1993; Back Pain 1994; Bigos 1994):

   A.   Rest and its duration

   B.   Exercise

   C.   Back school concept

   D.   Indications, concepts, and contraindications of manipulation

   E.   Value and indications for epidural steroids

   F.   Indications, types, and value of orthotic devices such as corset, brace, and cast

   G.   Indications for traction, types, and method of prescribing

       1.   Pelvic
       2.   Gravity

   H.   Medications: indications, value, and dosage

       1.   Nonsteroidal anti-inflammatory drugs
       2.   Muscle relaxants
       3.   Antidepressants
       4.   Analgesics

VI.   Know the indications for surgical intervention for low back pain (Mixter and Barr 1934; Spangfort 1972; Loeser 1990; Loeser 1991; Nachemson 1992; Turner 1992; Bigos 1994).

   A.   Be familiar with the signs and symptoms of the cauda equina syndrome.

   B.   Know how to recognize progressive neurological deficits and understand the implication for therapy.

   C.   Be able to differentiate various surgical procedures including laminectomy, diskectomy, nuclectomy, foraminotomy, and fusion.

   D.   Know the indications for and outcomes data for lumbar spine fusion and discectomy.

VII.   Know the etiologies of failed back surgery syndrome (Buront et al.1981; Loeser 1990; Frymoyer 1993).

VIII.   Know the role of nerve blocks in the diagnosis and management of low back pain (Cailliet 1988; Loeser 1990).

IX.   Be aware of the indications and basic principles and know the outcomes of facet rhizolysis in the treatment of low back pain (Cailliet 1988; Loeser 1990).

X.   Know the indications, costs, benefits, potential risks, and complications of the various treatment strategies for acute and chronic low back pain (Spitzer 1987; Frymoyer and Cats-Baril 1991; Epidemiology Review 1994).

XI.   Know the complaints, physical findings, and laboratory confirmation of pseudoclaudication from spinal stenosis (Cailliet 1988; Loeser 1990).

XII.   Know the role of multidisciplinary pain management in the treatment of chronic low back pain (Loeser 1990).

XIII.   Know the work-related factors, sitting postures, and activities of daily living that may be important in the aggravation of low back pain (Cailliet 1988; Frymoyer 1993).

XIV.   Be familiar with the incidence and prevalence of low back pain and its economic consequences. Understand the lack of correlation between physical findings, imaging studies, pain and suffering, health care consumption, and disability (Frymoyer and Cats-Baril 1991; Loeser 1991; Back Pain 1994; Clinical Standards Advisory Group 1994).

REFERENCES

Back Pain: Report of a CSAG Committee on Back Pain, Her Majesty's Stationary Office, London, 1994.

Bigos, S., Bowyer, O., Braen, G., et al., Acute Low Back Problems in Adults, Clinical Practice Guideline No. 14, AHCPR Publication No. 95-0642, U.S. Department of Health and Human Services, Public Health Service, Agency for Health Care Policy and Research, Rockville, MD, 1994.

Borenstein, D.G. and Wiesel, S.W., Low Back Pain, W.B. Saunders Co., Philadelphia, 1989.

Bortz,W., The disuse syndrome, West. J. Med., 141 (1984) 691–694.

Burton, C.V., Kirkaldy-Willis, W.H., Yong-Hing, K. and Heithoff, K.B., Causes of failure of surgery on the lumbar spine, Clin. Orthop., 157 (1981) 191–199.

Cailliet, R., Low Back Pain Syndrome (4th ed.), F.A. Davis Co., Philadelphia, 1988.

Clinical Standards Advisory Group, Epidemiology Review: The Epidemiology and Cost of Low Back Pain, Her Majesty's Stationery Office, London, 1994.

Deyo, R.A., Rainville, J. and Kent, D.L., What can the history and physical limitation tell us about low back pain? JAMA, 268 (1992) 760–765.

Frymoyer, J.W., Quality: an international challenge to diagnosis and treatment of disorders of the lumbar spine, Spine, 18 (1993) 2147–2152.

Frymoyer, J.W. and Cats-Baril, W.L., An overview of the incidences and costs of low back pain, Ortho. Clin. North Am., 22 (1991) 263–271.

Hoffman, R.M., Wheeler, K.J. and Deyo, R.A., Surgery for herniated lumbar discs: a literature synthesis, J. Gen. Int. Med., 8 (1993) 487–496.

Loeser, J.D. (Ed.), Low back pain. In: Neurosurgery Clinics of North America, Vol. 2, W.B. Saunders, Philadelphia, 1991.

Loeser, J.D., Bigos, S.J., Fordyce, W.E. and Volinn, E.P., Low back pain. In: J.J. Bonica (Ed.), The Management of Pain (2nd ed.), Lea & Febiger, Philadelphia, 1990, pp. 1448–1483.

Marras, P.A., Lavender, S.A., Leurgans, S.E., Rajulu, S.L., Allread, W.G., Fathallah, F.A. and Ferguson, S.A., The role of dynamic three-dimensional trunk motion in occupationally related low back disorders: the effects of workplace factors, trunk position, and trunk motion characteristics on risk of injury, Spine, 18 (1993) 617–628.

Mixter,W.J. and Barr, J.S., Rupture of the intervertebral disc with involvement of the spinal canal, N. Engl. J. Med., 211 (1934) 210–214.

Nachemson, A.L., Newest knowledge of low back pain: a critical look, Clin. Orthop., 279 (1992) 8–20.

Spangfort, E.V., The lumbar disc herniation: a computer-aided analysis of 2,504 operations, Acta. Orthop. Scand., Suppl. 142 (1972) 1–95.

Spitzer, W.D., LeBlanc, F.E. and Dupries, M., Scientific approach to the assessment and management of activity-related spinal disorders, Spine, 12 (1987) S1–S59.

Turner, J.A., Ersek, M., Herron, L., Haselkorn, J., Kent, D., Ciol, M.A. and Deyo, R.A. Patient outcomes after lumbar spinal fusions, JAMA, 268 (1992) 907–911.

Waddell, G., A new clinical model for the treatment of low back pain, Spine, 12 (1987) 632–644.

Weber, H., Lumbar disc herniation: a controlled prospective study with ten years of observation, Spine, 8 (1983) 131–140.

Core Curriculum for Professional Education in Pain, edited by H.L. Fields, IASP Press, Seattle, © 1995.

19

Myofascial Pain

I. Prevalence and importance

    A. Realize that about 50% of men and women develop myofascial trigger points by the age of 19 (Sola et al. 1955), that trigger points can be a significant cause of pain in up to half of chronic pain clinic patients (Fricton et al. 1985; Fishbain et al. 1986), and in one-third of pain patients in a general medical practice (Skootsky et al. 1989).

    B. Know that myofascial mechanisms commonly contribute to pain in tension headaches (Travell and Simons 1983; Jaeger 1989), low back syndromes (Simons and Travell 1983; Travell and Simons 1983, 1992; Rachlin 1994), and other musculoskeletal diagnoses throughout the body, including bursitis, arthritis, tendinitis, and muscle tears (Travell and Simons 1983, 1992; Rosen 1993; Rachlin 1994).

II. Pathophysiology

    A. Be aware of the metabolic crisis hypothesis explaining myofascial trigger points (Simons 1993). Understand the role of nerve sensitization causing pain and tenderness (Fields 1987; Fischer 1994, 1995b; Mense 1994; Simons 1994).

    B. Be aware of the hypothesis that a myofascial trigger point contains multiple dysfunctional loci (Fischer 1995b) that are closely associated with myoneural junctions (Gerwin 1994; Simons 1995).

    C. Appreciate the common occurrence and neurophysiological basis of pain referred to and from muscle (Kraus 1970; Travell and Simons 1983, 1992; Fields 1987; Kraus 1988; Simons 1988, 1994; Bonica 1990; Gerwin 1994; Mense 1994).

III. Clinical characteristics

    A. Note the clinical importance of distinguishing myofascial pain defined in a general sense (Fischer 1995) and as specifically applied to trigger points (Travell and Simons 1983; Kraus 1991; Simons 1995).

    B. Be able to distinguish between active trigger points and latent trigger points (Kraus 1970; Travell and Simons 1983, 1992; Fischer 1995b).

    C. Be aware of the differences between *primary* trigger points due to trauma or chronic overload of the muscle (Kraus 1970, 1988, 1991; Travell and Simons 1983, 1992; Sola and Bonica 1990) and *secondary* trigger points that arise from primary trigger points (Simons 1988; Rosen 1993) or from extramuscular sources (Hackett 1958; Fields 1987; Bonica 1990; Rachlin 1994).

IV. Evaluation

    A. Know the common trigger points responsible for pain in the:

        1. Head and neck region (Travell and Simons 1983)
        2. Shoulders and upper limbs (Travell and Simons 1983)
        3. Low back syndromes (Simons and Travell 1983; Travell and Simons 1983, 1992; Rachlin 1994)
        4. Torso and hip pain (Travell and Simons 1992)
        5. Lower limbs (Travell and Simons 1992)

    B. Be able to (Kraus 1970, 1988, 1991; Travell and Simons 1983, 1992; Sola and Bonica 1990; Rachlin 1994):

        1. Perform a test for specific limitation of motion by individual muscles and for muscle strength.
        2. Identify a taut band and within it the highly localized spot of maximum tenderness that indicates the trigger point itself (Travell and Simons 1983; Simons 1988; Fischer 1995b).
        3. Elicit the patient's myofascial pain complaint by pressure on the trigger point (Travell and Simons 1983; Fischer 1994; Njoo 1994; Fischer 1995b).

    C. Know that myofascial syndromes can become aggravated and perpetuated by other injuries and conditions (Travell and Simons 1983, 1992).

    D. Learn to distinguish fibromyalgia, which is a generalized condition, from myofascial pain, which is a group of local or regional pain syndromes. Recognize treatable myofascial components in fibromyalgia (Simons 1988; Rachlin 1994).

    E. Learn to distinguish muscle spasm affecting the entire muscle (Kraus 1988; Bonica 1990; Kraus 1991) from the taut band associated with trigger points (Travell and Simons 1983; Fischer 1987; 1995b; Simons 1988; Fischer 1995b). Also, differentiate emotional muscle tension and muscle stiffness (Kraus 1970, 1988, 1991) from trigger points (Travell and Simons 1983).

V. Treatment

    A. Understand that acute myofascial pain syndromes caused by trigger points are responsive to immediate treatment but may become difficult to manage when allowed to develop chronicity (Kraus 1970; Kraus 1988, 1991; Travell and Simons 1992).

    B. Learn the different therapeutic approaches including: spray and passive stretch (Travell and Simons 1983, 1992; Simons 1988), spray and active limbering (relaxation) exercises (Kraus 1970, 1988, 1991; Deyo 1990), postisometric relaxation (Travell and Simons 1992; Fischer 1995b), and reciprocal inhibition (Travell and Simons 1992; Fischer1995b), massage, trigger point compression, and trigger point injections to relieve myofascial pain (Frost et al. 1980; Travell and Simons 1983, 1992; Jaeger and Skootsky 1987; Garvey et al. 1989; Sola and Bonica 1990; Fischer et al. 1993; Hong 1994; Rachlin 1994; Fischer 1995a,b).

    C. Appreciate the importance of measuring changes in range of motion, pressure-pain thresholds by algometry (Fischer 1987, 1990, 1994; Fischer et al. 1993), and visual analog scale pain ratings to diagnose and record the progress of patients with chronic myofascial pain (Travell and Simons 1983, 1992; Fischer 1987, 1990, 1994; Jaeger 1989; Sola and Bonica 1990; Kraus 1991; Mense 1994).

D. Know the value of eliciting the local twitch response when injecting trigger points (Hong 1994; Fischer 1995a,b).

E. Be aware of the importance of a home exercise program, including stretch (Travell and Simons 1983, 1992), limbering (Kraus 1970, 1988; Deyo 1990; Rachlin 1994), reciprocal inhibition (Travell and Simons 1983, 1992; Fischer 1995b), and postisometric relaxation (Travell and Simons 1992) for treatment and prevention of myofascial pain syndromes.

REFERENCES

Bonica, J.J. (Ed.), The Management of Pain, Lea & Febiger, Philadelphia, 1990.

Deyo, R.A., A controlled trial of transcutaneous electrical nerve stimulation (TENS) and exercise for chronic low back pain. N. Engl. J. Med., 322 (1990) 1627–1634.

Fields, H.L., Pain, McGraw-Hill Book Co., New York, 1987.

Fischer, A.A., Pressure threshold measurement for diagnosis of myofascial pain and evaluation of treatment results, Clin. J. Pain, 2 (1987a) 207–214.

Fischer, A.A., Clinical use of tissue compliance meter for documentation of soft tissue pathology, Clin. J. Pain, 3 (1987b) 23–30.

Fischer, A.A., Application of pressure algometry in manual medicine, J. Manual Med., 5 (1990) 145–150.

Fischer, A.A., Commentary to Byrn, C., Olsson, I., Falkheden, L., Lindh, M., Hostereg, U., Fogelberg, M., Linder, L., Bunketorp, O., Subcutaneous sterile water injections for chronic neck and shoulder pain following whiplash injuries, Lancet, 341 (1993) 470.

Fischer, A.A., Pressure algometry (dolorimetry) in the differential diagnosis of muscle pain. In: E.S. Rachlin (Ed.), Myofascial Pain and Fibromyalgia, Trigger Point Management, Mosby, St. Louis (1994) pp. 121–141.

Fischer, A.A., Trigger point injection. In: T.A. Lennard (Ed.), Physiatric Procedures in Clinical Practice, Hanley & Belfus, Philadelphia, 1995a, pp. 28–35.

Fischer, A.A., Local injections in pain management: trigger point needling with infiltration and somatic blocks. In: S.M. Weinstein (Ed.), Physical Medicine and Rehabilitation Clinics of North America, W.B. Saunders, Philadelphia, 1995b.

Fishbain, D.A., Goldberg, M., Meagher, B.R., Steele, R. and Rosomoff, H., Male and female chronic pain patients categorized by DSM-III psychiatric diagnostic criteria, Pain, 26 (1986) 181–197.

Fricton, J.R., Kroening, R., Haley, D. and Siegert, R., Myofascial pain syndrome of the head and neck: a review of clinical characteristics of 164 patients, Oral Surg. Oral Med. Oral Path., 60 (1985) 615–623.

Frost, F.A., Jessen, B. and Siggaard-Andersen, J., A control, double-blind comparison of mepivacaine injection versus saline injection for myofascial pain, Lancet i, (1980) 499–500.

Garvey, T.A., Marks, M.R. and Wiesel, S.W., A prospective, randomized, double-blind evaluation of trigger-point injection therapy for low-back pain, Spine, 14 (1989) 962–964.

Gerwin, R.D., Neurobiology of the myofascial trigger point, In: Fibromyalgia and Myofascial Pain Syndromes, A.T. Massi (Ed.), Bailliere's Clinical Rheumatology, 8(4), Bailliere Tindall, London, 1994, pp. 747–762.

Hackett, G.S., Ligament and tendon relaxation treated by prolotherapy, 3rd ed., Thomas, Springfield, IL, 1958, pp. 27–36, 70.

Hong, C.-Z., Lidocaine injection versus dry needling to myofascial trigger point, Am. J. Phys. Med. Rehabil., 73 (1994) 256–263.

Jaeger, B., Are "cervicogenic" headaches due to myofascial pain and cervical spine dysfunction? Cephalalgia, 9 (1989) 157–164.

Jaeger, B. and Skootsky, S.A., Double-blind, controlled study of different myofascial trigger point injection techniques, Pain, 4 (suppl) (1987) S292.

Kraus, H., Clinical Treatment of Back and Neck Pain, McGraw Hill, New York, 1970.

Kraus, H., Diagnosis and Treatment of Muscle Pain, Quintessence Publishing Co., Chicago, 1988.

Kraus, H., Fischer, A.A., Diagnosis and treatment of myofascial pain, Mt. Sinai J. Med., 58 (1991) 235–239.

Mense, S, Referral of muscle pain: new aspects, APS Journal, 3 (1994) 1–9.

Njoo, K.H., The occurrence and inter-rater reliability of myofascial trigger points in the quadratus lumborum and gluteus medius: a prospective study in non-specific low back pain patients and controls in general practice, Pain, 58 (1994) 317–323.

Rachlin, E.S., Trigger points. In: E.S. Rachlin (Ed.), Myofascial Pain and Fibromyalgia, Mosby, St. Louis, 1994.

Rosen, N.B., Myofascial pain: the great mimicker and potentiator of other diseases in the performing artist, Md. Med. J., 42 (1993) 261–266.

Simons, D.G., Myofascial pain syndromes due to trigger points. In: J. Goodgold (Ed.), Rehabilitation Medicine, C.V. Mosby, St. Louis, 1988, pp. 686–723.

Simons, D.G., Referred phenomena of myofascial trigger points, In: L. Vecchiet, D. Albe-Fessard, U. Lindblom and M.A. Giamberardino (Eds.), New Trends in Referred Pain and Hyperalgesia, Pain Research and Clinical Management, No. 27, Elsevier Science Publishers, Amsterdam, 1993, pp. 341–357.

Simons, D.G., Neurophysiological basis of pain caused by trigger points, APS Journal, 3 (1994) 17–19.

Simons, D.G., Myofascial pain syndrome: one term but two concepts; a new understanding, J. Musculoskel. Pain, 3 (1995) 7–13.

Simons, D.G. and Travell, J.G., Myofascial origins of low back pain, Parts 1,2,3, Postgrad. Med., 73 (1983) 66–108.

Sola, A.E., Rodenberger, M.L. and Gettys, B.B., Incidence of hypersensitive areas in posterior shoulder muscles, Am. J. Phys. Med., 34 (1955) 585–590.

Sola, A.E., Bonica JJ: Myofascial pain syndromes. In: The Management of Pain, J.J. Bonica (Ed.), 2nd ed., Lea & Febiger, Philadelphia, 1990, pp. 352–367.

Skootsky, S.A., Jaeger, B. and Oye, R.K., Prevalence of myofascial pain in general internal medicine practice, West. J. Med., 151 (1989) 157–160.

Travell, J.G. and Simons, D.G., Myofascial Pain and Dysfunction: The Trigger Point Manual, Vol. 1, Williams & Wilkins, Baltimore, 1983.

Travell, J.G. and Simons, D.G., Myofascial Pain and Dysfunction: The Trigger Point Manual, The Lower Extremities, Vol. 2, Williams & Wilkins, Baltimore, 1992.

Core Curriculum for Professional Education in Pain, edited by H.L. Fields, IASP Press, Seattle, © 1995.

20

Neuropathic Pain

I. Know the common clinical characteristics of neuropathic pain (Sunderland 1978a,b; Wynn Parry 1980; Payne 1986; Fields 1987; Schwartzman and McLellan 1987; Portenoy 1989; Boivie 1994; Scadding 1994).

   A. Know the common symptoms associated with neuropathic pain (e.g., continuous burning pain referred to skin, paroxysmal [electric shock-like] pain, allodynia, radiating dysesthesias, and paresthesias).

   B. Know the common signs associated with neuropathic pain (e.g., sensory loss, weakness, autonomic changes, and trophic changes).

   C. Be aware of the clinical settings in which neuropathic pain occurs (e.g., peripheral nerve injury such as that occurring with surgical and traumatic amputations or soft tissue injuries, spinal cord injuries, stroke, cancer, acquired immune deficiency syndrome, diabetes, and herpes zoster).

II. Know the proposed pathological mechanisms of neuropathic pain (Bennett 1994; Devor 1994; Dickenson 1994; Fields and Rowbotham 1994; Jänig and McLachlan 1994; Perl 1994).

   A. In the periphery:

      1. Know the abnormal characteristics of primary afferent axonal sprouts ending in a neuroma (e.g., spontaneous discharge, ectopic mechanosensitivity, or acquired responsiveness to norepinephrine).
      2. Understand the proposed role in spontaneous discharge of sodium channel accumulation in the terminal membrane of neuroma sprouts.
      3. Understand the proposed role of acquired norepinephrine responsiveness in intact C-nociceptor terminals whose axons travel in a damaged nerve.
      4. Be aware of the potential role of irritation and inflammation of the nociceptor innervation of the nerve sheath.

   B. For the central nervous system:

      1. Understand the proposed role of N-methyl-D-aspartate (NMDA) receptor-mediated hyperexcitability in the spinal cord dorsal horn.
      2. Understand how spinal cord neuron hyperexcitability can account for pain that spreads beyond the innervation territory of a damaged peripheral nerve.
      3. Understand that a persistent source of nociceptor drive may dynamically maintain hyperexcitability in central neurons.
      4. Understand that spinal cord neurons may display abnormally increased activity when they lose their primary afferent innervation.

III. Know the following common neuropathic pain syndromes, including their clinical features, supporting laboratory and radiographic findings, and proposed pathology (Sunderland 1978a; Bennett 1994; Merskey and Bogduk 1994; Scadding 1994)

A. The major types of painful mononeuropathies (including peripheral mononeuropathies, plexopathies, and radiculopathies) (Dubuisson 1994; Scadding 1994).

1. Syndromes related to compression of peripheral nerves or nerve roots (e.g., lumbar and cervical radiculopathies and meralgia paresthetica)
2. Syndromes related to inflammation of peripheral nerves (e.g., acute herpetic neuralgia and acute inflammatory demyelinating neuropathy)
3. Syndromes related to ischemia/infarction of peripheral nerves (e.g., diabetic mononeuropathies)
4. Painful mononeuropathies of the orofacial region (e.g., trigeminal neuralgia)
5. Syndromes associated with neuroma formation (e.g., stump pain and postmastectomy pain)
6. Causalgia (complex regional pain syndrome, type II)

B. Painful polyneuropathies (Scadding 1994)

1. Be aware of the clinical presentation associated with painful polyneuropathy (e.g., burning feet).
2. Be aware of the differential diagnosis for common disorders associated with painful polyneuropathy (e.g., diabetes, vitamin deficiency, drug-induced [e.g., cancer chemotherapy-induced and AIDS-related]).

C. Know the clinical characteristics of postherpetic neuralgia and current concepts on its treatment and pathophysiology (Watson 1993; Fields and Rowbotham 1994).

D. Know the clinical characteristics of phantom pain and be able to differentiate it from other phantom sensations and from stump pain (Sunderland 1978a,b).

E. Know the clinical characteristics of pain from brachial plexus avulsion (Wynn Parry 1980).

F. Understand the concept of sympathetically maintained pain (SMP) (Payne 1986; Campbell et al 1992; Jänig and Koltzenberg 1992; Blumberg and Jänig 1994; Jänig and McLachlan 1994; Perl 1994).

1. Be aware of the current debate on how SMP can be diagnosed with local anesthetic blocks, Bier blocks with sympatholytic agents, and i.v. infusion with phentolamine.
2. Understand that SMP may be involved in several types of chronic neuropathic pain syndromes.
3. Know the clinical characteristics of reflex sympathetic dystrophy (RSD; complex regional pain syndrome, type III).

a. Know the controversial status of SMP as a necessary component of RSD diagnosis.
b. Understand the roles that X-ray, bone scan, autonomic testing, and thermography play in RSD diagnosis.
c. Understand that RSD evolves through different stages.

IV. Know the therapeutic interventions applied in neuropathic pain (Fields 1987; Portenoy 1989; Boivie 1994; Fields and Liebeskind 1994; Fields and Rowbotham 1994).

A. Know pharmacological approaches typically used for continuous neuropathic pain of all types.

1. Know specific agents and syndromes for which data from controlled clinical trials establish efficacy (e.g., amitriptyline in postherpetic neuralgia and diabetic neuropathy).
2. Know agents for which substantial anecdotal evidence exists for efficacy in continuous neuropathic pain (e.g., other tertiary amine tricyclics).
3. Know those drugs for which there is limited anecdotal evidence on efficacy for continuous neuropathic pain (e.g., selected neuroleptics).

B. Know drugs typically used in the treatment of sympathetically mediated pain and be aware of the limited data in support of their use (e.g., corticosteroids, phenoxybenzamine, prazosin, guanethidine, and clonidine).

C. Know those drugs typically used in the treatment of lancinating neuropathic pains.

1. Know those drugs and pain syndromes for which data from controlled studies establish efficacy (e.g., carbamazepine, diphenylhydantoin, baclofen, and mexiletine in trigeminal neuralgia).
2. Know those drugs for which there is limited controlled anecdotal evidence supporting efficacy (e.g., phenytoin, valproate, mexiletine, and clonazepam).

D. Be aware of the limited data supporting the use of nonsteroidal anti-inflammatory drugs and opioid analgesics in the management of neuropathic pain.

E. Know the role of regional approaches in the management of neuropathic pain. Be aware of the indications, techniques and potential complications of sympathetic blockade in syndromes believed to be sympathetically mediated pain.

1. Know the different types of local sympathetic blocks.
2. Know the indications, advantages and disadvantages, and drugs and techniques employed in regional intravenous blockade.
3. Understand the limited role of sympathectomy in patients who respond to temporary sympathetic blocks.
4. Be aware of the methods employed to document effective regional sympathetic block (e.g., thermography and laser Doppler studies).
5. Be aware of the existence, possible causes, and treatment of postsympathectomy pain (Perl 1994).

F. Know the role of surgical approaches to pain management in patients with neuropathic pain.

1. Be aware of the role of peripheral procedures in selected patients with specific pain syndromes (e.g., decompression of entrapped peripheral nerves or controlled trigeminal gangliolysis in trigeminal neuralgia).
2. Be aware of the anecdotal data contraindicating neurolytic procedures in neuropathic pain.
3. Be aware of the data suggesting the potential efficacy of dorsal root entry zone lesions in selected patients with specific pain syndromes (e.g., avulsion of the brachial plexus, or pain following spinal cord injury).

G. Be aware of neurostimulatory approaches to the management of neuropathic pain.

1. Be aware of the variability in response to transcutaneous electrical nerve stimulation and the multiple methods that can be employed.
2. Be aware of the data supporting and the data refuting the value of acupuncture.

3. Be aware of neurostimulation techniques.

    a. Understand the limited role played by percutaneous electrical nerve stimulation.
    b. Be aware of the data supporting and refuting the value of dorsal column stimulation.
    c. Be aware of the data supporting and refuting the value of deep brain stimulation.

H. Know the utility of psychiatric approaches to neuropathic pain management.

1. Understand the fundamental importance of physical therapy in treatment for some neuropathic disorders (e.g., reflex sympathetic dystrophy and postherpetic neuralgia).
2. Know the analgesic potential of orthoses and prostheses in selected patients with particular pain syndromes (e.g., a prosthesis for a patient with stump pain).
3. Have knowledge of a multidisciplinary approach to the patient with pain and related disabilities secondary to neuropathic lesion, and understand the importance of maintained function as a goal equal in importance to the goal of pain relief.

REFERENCES

Bennett, G.J., Neuropathic pain. In: P.D. Wall and R. Melzack (Eds.), Textbook of Pain, 3rd ed., Churchill Livingstone, Edinburgh, 1994, pp. 201–224.

Blumberg, H. and Jänig, W., Clinical manifestations of reflex sympathetic dystrophy and sympathetically maintained pain. In: P.D. Wall and R. Melzack (Eds.), Textbook of Pain, 3rd ed., Churchill Livingstone, Edinburgh, 1994, pp. 685–698.

Boivie, J., Central pain. In: P.D. Wall and R. Melzack (Eds.), Textbook of Pain, 3rd ed., Churchill Livingstone, Edinburgh, 1994, pp. 871–902.

Campbell, J.N., Meyer, R.A. and Raja, S.N., Is nociceptor activation by alpha-1 adrenoreceptors the culprit in sympathetically maintained pain? APS Journal , 13 (1992) 334–350.

Devor, M., The pathophysiology of damaged peripheral nerve. In: P.D. Wall and R. Melzack (Eds.), Textbook of Pain, 3rd ed., Churchill Livingstone, Edinburgh, 1994, pp. 79–100.

Dickenson, A.H., NMDA receptor antagonists as analgesics. In: H.L. Fields and J.C. Liebeskind (Eds.), Pharmacological Approaches to the Treatment of Chronic Pain: New Concepts and Critical Issues, Progress in Pain Research and Management, Vol. 1, IASP Press, Seattle, 1994, pp. 173–187.

Dubuisson, D., Nerve root damage and arachnoiditis. In: P.D. Wall and R. Melzack (Eds.), Textbook of Pain, 3rd ed., Churchill Livingstone, Edinburgh, 1994, pp. 711–735.

Fields, H.L., Pain, McGraw-Hill, New York, 1987.

Fields, H.L. and Liebeskind, J.C. (Eds.), Pharmacological Approaches to the Treatment of Chronic Pain: New Concepts and Critical Issues, Progress in Pain Research and Management, Vol. 1, IASP Press, Seattle, 1994.

Fields, H.L. and Rowbotham, M.C., Multiple mechanisms of neuropathic pain: a clinical perspective. In: G.F. Gebhart, D.L. Hammond and T.S. Jensen (Eds.), Proceedings of the 7th World Congress on Pain, Progress in Pain Research and Management, Vol. 2, IASP Press, Seattle, 1994, pp. 437–454.

Jänig, W. and Koltzenburg, M., Possible ways of sympathetic-afferent interactions. In: W. Jänig and R.F. Schmidt (Eds.), Pathophysiological Mechanisms of Reflex Sympathetic Dystrophy, VCH, Weinheim, 1992, pp. 213–243.

Jänig, W. and McLachlan, E.M., The role of modification in noradrenergic peripheral pathways after nerve lesions in the generation of pain. In: H.L. Fields and J.C. Liebeskind (Eds.), Pharmacological Approaches to the Treatment of Chronic Pain: New Concepts and Critical Issues, Progress in Pain Research and Management, Vol. 1, Seattle, IASP Press, 1994, pp. 101–128.

Merskey, H. and Bogduk, N. (Eds.), Classification of Chronic Pain: Descriptions of Chronic Pain Syndromes and Definitions of Pain Terms, 2nd ed., IASP Press, Seattle, 1994.

Payne, R., Neuropathic pain syndromes, with special reference to causalgia and reflex sympathetic dystrophy, Clin. J. Pain, 2 (1986) 59–73.

Perl, E.R., A reevaluation of mechanisms leading to sympathetically related pain. In: H.L. Fields and J.C. Liebeskind (Eds.), Pharmacological Approaches to the Treatment of Chronic Pain: New Concepts and Critical Issues, Progress in Pain Research and Management, Vol. 1, IASP Press, Seattle, 1994, pp. 129–150.

Portenoy, R.K. (Ed.), Pain: Mechanisms and Syndromes, Neurologic Clinics, W.B. Saunders., Philadelphia, 1989.

Scadding, J.W., Peripheral neuropathies. In: P.D. Wall and R. Melzack (Eds.), Textbook of Pain, 3rd ed., Churchill Livingstone, Edinburgh, 1994, pp. 667–683.

Schwartzman, R.J. and McLellan, J., Reflex Sympathetic Dystrophy, a review, Arch. Neurol., 44 (1987) 555–561.

Sunderland, S., The painful sequelae of injuries to peripheral nerves. In: S. Sunderland, Nerves and Nerve Injuries, 2nd ed., Churchill Livingstone, Edinburgh, 1978a, pp. 377–420.

Sunderland, S., Stump pain and abnormal sensory phenomena superimposed on the phantom state. In: S. Sunderland, Nerves and Nerve Injuries, 2nd ed., Churchill Livingstone, Edinburgh, 1978b, pp. 433–447.

Watson, C.P.N., Herpes Zoster and Postherpetic Neuralgia, Elsevier, Amsterdam, 1993.

Wynn Parry, C.B., Pain in avulsion lesions of the brachial plexus, Pain, 9 (1980) 41–53.

Core Curriculum for Professional Education in Pain, edited by H.L. Fields, IASP Press, Seattle, © 1995.

21

Headache

I. Know the anatomy and physiology relevant to headache.

    A. Pain-sensitive structures of the head
    B. Physiology of trigeminal nociception
    C. Cephalic vascular system and its innervation

II. Be aware of major hypotheses about mechanisms of headache.

    A. Peripheral nociception, including the concepts of perivascular neuroinflammation and dilatation of cerebral arteries
    B. Central dysmodulation
    C. 5-hydroxytryptamine involvement
    D. Myofascial mechanisms

III. Be able to record a systematic case history of headache and to use a headache diary. Be able to differentiate multiple headache disorders in a single patient. Be able to elicit and understand the clinical significance of the following:

    A. Duration and frequency of attacks
    B. Severity, quality, location, and referral of pain
    C. Age, time, and mode of onset
    D. Aura symptoms (immediately preceding headache)
    E. Associated symptoms (e.g., nausea, phonophobia, photophobia)
    F. Precipitating and aggravating factors
    G. Relieving factors
    H. Psychosocial stress
    F. Present or previous traumas and diseases
    G. Family history

IV. Know how to select and execute an appropriate examination on the basis of case history.

    A. General physical examination
    B. Neurological examination
    C. Pericranial palpation

V. Be aware of the classification of headache disorders. Be aware of the internationally accepted diagnostic criteria for the following headache disorders:

    A. Migraine with and without aura
    B. Tension-type headache
    C. Cluster headache

VI.   Know the indications for further investigation of headache.

VII. Understand the physical, psychological, and social factors that may contribute to headache, and know the importance of counseling and other nonpharmacological means of treatment.

VIII. Be able to use the following pharmacological agents appropriately, and be aware of possible alternatives.

A. Acetaminophen, acetylsalicylic acid, and other nonsteroidal anti-inflammatory drugs (NSAIDs) for acute headaches (and migraine attacks), and their possible combination with antiemetics and sedatives
B. Ergotamine and sumatriptan for acute attacks of migraine
C. Oxygen inhalation and sumatriptan injections for acute attacks of cluster headache
D. Beta-blockers for prophylaxis of migraine
E. Verapamil for prophylaxis of cluster headache

IX.   Know, for the above-mentioned pharmacological agents:

A. Rationale for use
B. Appropriate dosage and route of administration
C. Effects and side effects
D. Degree of documentation by controlled clinical trials
E. Risk of inappropriate use in daily or near-daily headache

REFERENCES

Headache Classification Committee of the International Headache Society, Classification and diagnostic criteria for headache disorders, cranial neuralgias and facial pain, Cephalalgia, 9 (Suppl.) (1988) 120–196.

Kudrow, L., Cluster Headache: Mechanisms and Treatment, Oxford University Press, Oxford, 1980.

Lance, J.W., Mechanism and Management of Headache, 5th ed., Butterworths, London, 1993.

Olesen, J. and Edvinsson, L. (Eds.), Basic Mechanisms of Headache, Elsevier, Amsterdam, 1988.

Olesen, J., Tfelt-Hansen, P. and Welch, K.M.A., The Headaches, Raven Press, New York, 1993.

Raskin, N.H., Headache, 2nd ed., Churchill Livingstone, Edinburgh, 1988.

Core Curriculum for Professional Education in Pain, edited by H.L. Fields, IASP Press, Seattle, © 1995.

22

Rheumatological Aspects of Pain

I. Epidemiology of musculoskeletal pain (Maddison et al. 1993; Cassidy and Petty 1995)

A. Know that chronic musculoskeletal pain is common and affects all age groups, particularly children ages three to five; frequency increases with age (Goodman and McGrath 1992; Magni et al. 1990; Badley et al. 1994).

B. Know that rheumatic disease is the preeminent cause of morbidity and health care service usage. Know that rheumatic disease is a major cause of disability, and musculoskeletal pain is an important factor associated with disability (Badley et al. 1994,1995).

C. Be aware that there are gender differences among types and frequencies of musculoskeletal pain.

II. Pathophysiology of musculoskeletal pain (Maddison et al. 1993)

A. Be familiar with the afferent and spinal mechanisms of joint and muscle pain (Mense 1993; Schaible and Grubb 1993).

B. Know that efferent neuronal mechanisms may contribute to joint inflammation (Schaible and Grubb 1993).

C. Know that inflammatory mediators, including neuropeptides and cytokines, are involved in the generation and persistence of inflammatory causes of musculoskeletal pain (Koch et al. 1995).

D. Be aware that pain from muscle and joint pathology is frequently referred to other structures.

III. Psychosocial aspects of musculoskeletal pain. Understand that musculoskeletal pain perception results from an interaction between psychosocial factors and joint inflammation and damage (Magni et al. 1990,1993; Smedstad et al. 1995; Wolfe et al. 1995).

IV. Classification of musculoskeletal diseases (Maddison et al. 1993; Cassidy and Petty 1995)

A. Recognize that there are three major groupings of musculoskeletal disease with unique clinical features and pain manifestations:

1. Soft-tissue
2. Noninflammatory joint disease
3. Inflammatory joint disease

B. Be aware that musculoskeletal pains occur commonly in children and that causes of pain in children differ from the causes of adult pains. Be aware that arthropathies manifest differently in children and adults (Cassidy and Petty 1993; Southwood and Malleson 1993).

C. Be familiar with the common arthropathies: osteoarthritis, rheumatoid arthritis, spondyloarthropathy. Know the different patterns of joint involvement in these common arthropathies. Be aware that rheumatoid arthritis is more common in women, that osteoarthritis has an equal sex distribution, and that spondyloarthropathy is more common in men (Maddison et al. 1993).

D. Be familiar with the concept of myofascial pain and the fibromyalgia syndrome. Know that fibromyalgia may be associated with other pain complaints (headaches, irritable bowel or bladder pain, or dysmenorrhea), and it may represent a generalized abnormality of pain modulation (Wolfe et al. 1990; Csillag 1992; Mufson and Regestein 1993).

E. Know that osteoporosis is a common cause of painful disability (Nevitt 1994).

V. Assessment of disease activity and severity (Glossary Committee 1988; Resnick and Niwayama 1988; Maddison et al. 1993)

A. Be able to assess joint range of motion, muscle strength, and joint tenderness and to recognize joint inflammation/deformity (Hoppenfeld 1976).

B. Be able to radiographically distinguish abnormal bones and joints (Resnick and Niwayama 1988).

C. Know how to use acute phase reactants (erythrocyte sedimentation rate, C-reactive protein, or platelet count) to monitor disease activity.

D. Know that joint fluid can be used to help differentiate various causes of inflammation.

E. Understand that multiple instruments are available to evaluate and quantify different aspects of musculoskeletal disease (Glossary Committee 1988).

1. Joint counts (Cooperating Clinics 1965; Ritchie et al. 1968)
2. Functional and Activities of Daily Living Measure (Steinbrocker et al. 1949)
3. Multidimensional health status instruments: Arthritis Impact Measurement Scales, and Health Assessment Questionnaire (Fries et al. 1980; Meenan et al. 1980; Glossary Committee 1988)

F. Know that pain is one of the main concerns of arthritis patients; self-reported pain has been recommended as a core endpoint measure in rheumatoid arthritis, and this measure is sensitive to change in arthritis activity (Tugwell and Boers 1993; Affleck et al. 1991; Anderson and Chernoff 1993).

G. Know that extant instruments for assessment of pain in children are not yet developmentally appropriate (Glossary Committee 1988; De Inocencio and Lovell 1993; also see Chapters 6 and 28).

VI. Treatment of musculoskeletal pain (Melvin 1989; Maddison et al. 1993; Cassidy and Petty 1995)

A. Know the role of local pain control measures—i.e., heat, cold, passive and active movement, and splints (Melvin 1989; Schlapbach and Gerber 1991).

B. Be aware of the risks and benefits of rest and exercise (Minor et al. 1989; Malmivaara et al. 1995).

C. Understand the role of nonsteroidal anti-inflammatory drugs compared with simple analgesics. Know indications for, routes of administration of, and adverse effects of:

1. Corticoids
2. Methotrexate, antimalarials, sulfasalazine gold
3. Azathioprine and cyclophosphamide

D. Be aware of compliance issues in management of chronic rheumatic pain.

E. Understand that many rheumatic diseases require a multidisciplinary team management approach.

REFERENCES

Affleck, G., Tennen, H., Urrows, S. and Higgins, P., Individual differences in the day-to-day experience of chronic pain: a prospective daily study of rheumatoid arthritis patients, Health Psychol., 10 (1991) 419–426.

Anderson, J.J. and Chernoff, M.C., Sensitivity to change of rheumatoid arthritis clinical trial outcome measures, J. Rheumatol., 20 (1993) 535–537.

Badley, E.M., Rasooly, I. and Webster, G.K., Relative importance of musculoskeletal disorders as a cause of chronic health problems, disability, and health care utilization: findings from the 1990 Ontario Health Survey, J. Rheumatol., 21 (1994) 505–514.

Badley, E.M., Webster, G.K. and Rasooly, I., The impact of musculoskeletal disorders in the population: are they just aches and pains? Findings from the 1990 Ontario Health Survey, J. Rheumatol., 22 (1995) 733–739.

Cassidy, J.T. and Petty, R.E. (Eds.), Textbook of Pediatric Rheumatology, 3rd ed., W.B. Saunders, Philadelphia, 1995.

Cooperating Clinics Committee of the American Rheumatism Association, A seven-day variability study of 499 patients with peripheral rheumatoid arthritis, Arthritis Rheum., 8 (1965) 302–334.

Csillag, C., Fibromyalgia: the Copenhagen declaration, Lancet, 340 (1992) 663–664.

De Inocencio, J. and Lovell, D.J., Clinical and functional monitoring, outcome measures and prognosis of juvenile chronic arthritis. In: T.R. Southwood and P.N. Malleson (Eds.), Arthritis in Children and Adolescents, Baillière Tindall, London, 1993, pp. 769–801.

Fries, J.F., Spitz, P., Kraines, R.G. and Holman, H., Measurement of patient outcome in arthritis, Arthritis Rheum., 23 (1980) 137–145.

Glossary Committee of the American College of Rheumatology, Dictionary of the Rheumatic Diseases, Vol. III, Health Status Measurement, American College of Rheumatology, Atlanta, 1988.

Goodman, J.E. and McGrath, P.J., The epidemiology of pain in children and adolescents: a review, Pain, 46 (1992) 247–264.

Hoppenfeld, S., Physical Examination of the Spine and Extremities, Appleton-Century-Crofts, Norwalk, 1976.

Koch, A.E., Kunkel, S.L. and Strieter, R.M., Cytokines in rheumatoid arthritis., J. Invest. Med., 43 (1995) 28–38.

Maddison, P.J., Isenberg, D.A., Woo, P. and Glass, D.N. (Eds.), Oxford Textbook of Rheumatology, Oxford University Press, Oxford, 1993.

Magni, G., Caldieron, C., Rigatti-Luchini, S. and Merskey, H., Chronic musculoskeletal pain and depressive symptoms in the general population: an analysis of the First National Health and Nutrition Examination Survey data., Pain, 43 (1990) 299–307.

Magni, G., Marchetti, M., Moreschi, C., Merskey, H. and Rigatti-Luchini, S., Chronic musculoskeletal pain and depressive symptoms in the National Health and Nutrition Examination. I. Epidemiologic follow-up study, Pain, 53 (1993) 163–168.

Malmivaara, A., Hakkinen, U., Aro, T., Heinrichs, M.L., Koskenniemi, L., Kuosma, E., Lappi, S., Paloheimo, R. Servo, C., Vaaranen, V., et al., The treatment of low back pain: bed rest, exercises, or ordinary activity? N. Engl. J. Med., 332 (1995) 351–355.

Meenan, R.F., Gertman, P.M. and Mason, J.H., Measuring health status in arthritis: the Arthritis Impact Measurement Scales, Arthritis Rheum., 23 (1980) 146–152.

Melvin, J.L., Rheumatic Disease in the Adult and Child: Occupational Therapy and Rehabilitation, 3rd ed., F.A. Davis, Philadelphia, 1989.

Mense, S., Nociception from skeletal muscle in relation to clinical muscle pain, Pain, 54 (1993) 241–289.

Minor, M.A., Hewitt, J.E., Webel, R.R., Anderson, S.K. and Kay, D.R., Efficacy of physical conditioning exercise in patients with rheumatoid arthritis and osteoarthritis, Arthritis Rheum., 32 (1989) 1396–1405.

Mufson, M. and Regestein, Q.R., The spectrum of fibromyalgia disorders (editorial), Arthritis Rheum., 36 (1993) 647–649.

Nevitt, M.C., Epidemiology of osteoporosis, Rheum. Dis. Clin. North Am., 20 (1994) 535–559.

Resnick, D. and Niwayama, G., (Eds.), Diagnosis of Bone and Joint Disorders, 2nd ed., W.B. Saunders, Philadelphia, 1988.

Ritchie, D.M., Boyle, J.A., McInnes, J.M., Jasani, M.K., Dalakoj, T.G., Grieveson, P. and Buchanan, W.W., Clinical studies with an articular index for the assessment of joint tenderness in patients with rheumatoid arthritis, Quarterly Journal of Medicine, 37 (1968) 393–406.

Schaible, H. and Grubb, B.D., Afferent and spinal mechanisms of joint pain, Pain, 55 (1993) 5–54.

Schlapbach, P. and Gerber, N.J. (Eds.), Physiotherapy: Controlled Trials and Facts, Karger, Basel, Switzerland, 1991.

Smedstad, L.M., Vaglum, P., Kvien, T.K. and Torbjorn, M., The relationship between self-reported pain and sociodemographic variables, anxiety, and depressive symptoms in rheumatoid arthritis, J. Rheumatol., 22 (1995) 514–520.

Southwood, T.R. and Malleson, P.N. (Eds.), Arthritis in Children and Adolescents, Baillière Tindall, London, 1993.

Steinbrocker, O., Traeger, C.H. and Batterman, R.C., Therapeutic criteria in rheumatoid arthritis, JAMA, 140 (1949) 659–662.

Tugwell, P. and Boers, M., Developing consensus on preliminary core efficacy endpoints for rheumatoid arthritis clinical trials., J. Rheumatol., 20 (1993) 555–556.

Wolfe F., Smythe H.A., Yunus, M.B., Bennett. R.M., Bombardier, C., Goldenberg, D.L., Tugwell, P., Campbell, S.M., Abelels, M., Clark, P., et al., The American College of Rheumatology 1990 criteria for the classification of fibromyalgia. Report of the multicenter criteria committee, Arthritis Rheum., 33 (1990) 160–172.

Wolfe, F., Ross, K., Anderson, J., Russell, I.J. and Hebert, L., The prevalence and characteristics of fibromyalgia in the general population, Arthritis Rheum., 38 (1995) 19–28.

Core Curriculum for Professional Education in Pain, edited by H.L. Fields, IASP Press, Seattle, © 1995.

23

Cancer Pain

I. General principles (American Society of Clinical Oncology 1992; Cherny and Portenoy 1994a; Cleeland et al. 1994; Jacox et al. 1994; Twycross 1994)

    A. Understand that pain is experienced by more than one-third of cancer patients who are receiving active therapy and more than three-quarters of those with far advanced disease.

    B. Know that adequate pain relief can be achieved by 70–90% of cancer patients who receive optimal analgesic management.

    C. Recognize that pain management is a component of a broader therapeutic endeavor known as palliative care. Understand that palliative care is defined as the active, total care of the patient with life-threatening disease and provides an interdisciplinary model for the continuing management of quality-of-life concerns, including control of symptoms, maintenance of function, psychosocial and spiritual support for the patient and family, and comprehensive care at the end of life (World Health Organization 1992; Doyle et al. 1993).

    D. Understand the barriers to cancer pain treatment, including patient-related barriers, health care provider barriers, and health policy and reimbursement barriers. Recognize the importance of health care provider education in removing these barriers.

II. Evaluation of patients with cancer pain (Miser and Miser 1989; Gonzales et al. 1991; Patt 1993; Cherny and Portenoy 1994a; DeConno et al. 1994; Twycross 1994)

    A. Recognize the importance of the comprehensive assessment and understand that optimal pain management within the broader context of palliative care depends on detailed information about the pain itself, comorbid medical and psychosocial problems, premorbid and current physical and psychosocial functioning of the patient and family, goals of care, and other factors.

    B. Be aware that cancer pain is highly associated with structural pathology and that, consequently, definition of the extent of the disease and the nature of the specific underlying etiology of the pain are essential outcomes of the pain assessment (Gonzales et al. 1991).

    C. Understand that the comprehensive evaluation of cancer pain requires an accurate history, a physical and neurological examination, a review of laboratory and radiographic procedures, and possibly additional testing.

    D. Understand the importance of an accurate characterization of the pain or pains in terms of location, severity, quality, temporal factors, and provocative and palliative factors.

    E. Understand that the consistent use of a valid pain measurement scale (e.g., verbal categorical, numerical, visual analog) can help guide clinical decisions concerning additional assessment and therapy. Be aware of the need to use age-appropriate pain measurement approaches for children with cancer pain.

F. Recognize the significance of temporal patterns of pain (e.g., continuous, intermittent, acute inter-mittent pains superimposed on continuous pain) in terms of treatment decisions (e.g., use of sup-plemental "as-needed" doses of an opioid to treat "breakthrough pain"). Understand that rapidly escalating pain ("crescendo pain") is an emergency that requires prompt intervention.

G. Be aware that syndrome recognition is an essential outcome of the pain assessment (Cherny and Portenoy 1994a). Recognize that syndrome diagnosis can help guide the evaluation of cancer pain and provide information relevant to treatment and prognosis. Know the characteristics of common pain syndromes that are direct effects of a tumor, those that result from antineoplastic therapies, and those that result from factors unrelated to the disease or its treatment. Know the common oncologic emergencies that present with pain and be aware of the need for a prompt evaluation of these syn-dromes (e.g., back pain as a harbinger of epidural spinal cord compression).

H. Understand the importance of inferring a pathophysiological mechanism for each pain and the im-plications for therapy that such information suggests (Cherny and Portenoy 1994a). Be aware of the classification that distinguishes "nociceptive pains," which are believed to be sustained by continu-ing injury to somatic structures ("somatic pain") or visceral structures ("visceral pain"), from "neuropathic pains," which are believed to be sustained by abnormal processes in the peripheral or central nervous systems (including painful peripheral mononeuropathy and polyneuropathy; reflex sympathetic dystrophy or causalgia syndromes, some of which are sympathetically maintained pain; and deafferentation pain). Recognize that pain predominantly sustained by psychological factors appears to be rare in the cancer population, notwithstanding the importance of psychological factors in the expression and impact of the pain.

I. Recognize that an increase in pain intensity following a stable period should impel a new evaluation of the underlying etiology and pain syndrome.

J. Understand the assessment of factors other than the pain, including other physical symptoms (e.g., fatigue, nausea and constipation), coexistent psychological symptoms and psychiatric disorders (e.g., depression), functional status, family disturbances, social and familial support systems, medi-cal support systems, and financial resources. Recognize the importance of assessing the availability of primary antineoplastic therapies and of assessing the existence of other medical disorders (e.g., hypercalcemia).

II. Principles of cancer pain treatment (Miser and Miser 1989; World Health Organization 1992; Arbit 1993; Patt 1993; Cherny and Portenoy 1994b; Cleeland et al. 1994; Jacox et al. 1994; Twycross 1994)

A. Recognize that therapies for pain must be integrated into the oncologic management of the patient, which often includes both primary antineoplastic therapy intended to prolong life and the broader palliative care of the patient.

B. Recognize that treatments that ameliorate the underlying pathology may be useful in the manage-ment of cancer pain. Understand that these treatments comprise radiotherapy, pharmacotherapy (including chemotherapy, hormonal agents, and antibiotic therapy), and surgery. Know that the use of any primary therapy for analgesic purposes requires careful evaluation of its feasibility, risk ver-sus benefit, and appropriateness given the overriding goals of care.

C. Know that analgesic pharmacotherapy is the mainstay of cancer pain management and that most patients with cancer pain can be effectively managed with an optimal opioid regimen. Recognize the importance of expertise in opioid therapy for all practitioners who treat patients with cancer.

D. Recognize the importance of other therapeutic modalities for the treatment of cancer pain. Understand that many patients could achieve better pain control if opioid therapy were integrated with other analgesic modalities and that some patients, specifically those who are unable to achieve a favorable balance between opioid analgesia and side effects, require such an alternative approach for the major intervention. Know that alternative modalities comprise many anesthesiological approaches, neurostimulatory therapies, surgical interventions, physiatric treatments, and psychological approaches.

III. Pharmacological approaches to cancer pain (Miser and Miser 1989; World Health Organization 1992; Arbit 1993; Doyle et al. 1993; Patt 1993; Cherny and Portenoy 1994b; Eisenberg et al. 1994; Jacox et al. 1994; Twycross 1994)

A. Understand the "analgesic ladder" approach to drug selection and know the indications and dosing guidelines for the nonopioid analgesics, including acetaminophen (paracetamol) and the nonsteroidal anti-inflammatory drugs (step one); the opioids conventionally used orally for moderate pain, including codeine, oxycodone (when combined with a nonopioid analgesic in a single tablet), propoxyphene, hydrocodone, and dihydrocodeine (step two); and opioids conventionally used for severe cancer pain, including morphine, hydromorphone, oxycodone (as a single entity), levorphanol, methadone, fentanyl, and heroin (step three).

B. Understand the essential pharmacokinetics of opioid analgesics, including the relationships between kinetics and effects and the importance of active metabolites for some opioids (specifically morphine and meperidine).

C. Know the reasons that meperidine and drugs in the agonist-antagonist class of opioids are not preferred for cancer pain management.

D. Understand the rationale for oral administration whenever feasible.

E. Be familiar with the availability of, and indications for, other routes of opioid administration, including sublingual, rectal, transdermal, subcutaneous and intravenous (by repetitive administration, continuous infusion, patient controlled analgesia), intramuscular, epidural (by repetitive administration, continuous infusion, and patient controlled analgesia via a percutaneous catheter, an implanted subcutaneous portal, or an implanted pump), intrathecal, and intraventricular.

F. Know the appropriate dosing intervals: specifically, 3–4 hours for most opioids in most patients; sometimes longer intervals (every 6 hours or longer) when using methadone or buprenorphine, 8–12 hours with controlled release morphine, and 48–72 hours with the transdermal fentanyl system.

G. Understand the value of "around-the-clock" dosing but also be aware of the importance of supplemental "rescue" doses offered on an as-needed basis for pain exacerbations.

H. Understand the critical importance of dose titration to individualize opioid therapy. Know that dose titration is based on the principle that the dose should be increased until adequate analgesia occurs or intolerable and unmanageable side effects supervene. Recognize that the absolute dose is immaterial as long as a favorable balance between analgesia and side effects is maintained.

I. Understand the use of adjuvant drugs to manage common side effects, and the importance of side effect management in optimizing the response to opioid therapy. Be aware of dosing guidelines for laxatives (bulk, osmotic, and stimulant agents) and the techniques used for refractory constipation, including chronic therapy with lactulose or sorbitol, chronic bowel lavage, and oral naloxone. Be aware of the use of antiemetics for the treatment of opioid-induced nausea. Be aware of the use of psychostimulants for opioid-induced somnolence and cognitive impairment

J. Understand that the risk of respiratory depression is extremely low when opioid doses are gradually titrated and recognize that opioid-induced respiratory depression is always associated with slowed respirations and obtundation. Be aware that the occurrence of a new cardiopulmonary insult in a patient who is receiving opioids may produce respiratory depression that is, in part, naloxone-reversible, so that the response to naloxone is not evidence for a primary effect of the opioid.

K. Understand the concept of equianalgesic doses and the use of the equianalgesic dose table when switching from opioid to opioid or from one route of administration to another.

L. Understand the concept of tolerance and its importance in cancer pain management. Be aware of the data demonstrating that cancer patients with stable disease seldom escalate opioid dose. Be aware of anecdotal observations suggesting that patients who do escalate the opioid dose generally do so in the setting of a recurrent or progressive lesion.

M. Understand the concept of physical dependence and its implications for cancer pain management. Be aware of the need to prevent abstinence by tapering opioids prior to discontinuation of therapy and avoiding antagonist drugs, including agonist-antagonist opioids.

N. Understand that addiction is fundamentally a psychological and behavioral disorder characterized by loss of control over drug use, compulsive drug use, and continued drug use despite harm. Know that iatrogenic addiction during opioid treatment for cancer pain is almost never observed.

O. Understand the indications, pharmacological properties, and appropriate dosing guidelines for the so-called adjuvant analgesics, drugs with primary indications other than pain that may be coanalgesic in selected circumstances (Chapter 9) (Doyle et al. 1993; Cherny and Portenoy 1994b). Understand the use of the following drugs for cancer-related neuropathic pain: antidepressants, systemic (oral and intravenous) local anesthetics, anticonvulsants, corticosteroids, and miscellaneous drugs such as baclofen and clonidine. Understand the use of the following drugs for malignant bone pain: nonsteroidal anti-inflammatory drugs, corticosteroids, calcitonin, bisphosphonates, and radiopharmaceuticals (e.g., strontium-89). Understand the use of the following drugs for malignant bowel obstruction: corticosteroids, anticholinergic drugs (e.g., scopolamine), and octreotide.

IV. Anesthesiological approaches to cancer pain (Patt 1993)

A. Understand the indications, risks, and practical implications of intraspinal therapies for cancer pain, including epidural or intrathecal opioids or local anesthetics delivered by percutaneous or implanted systems.

B. Be aware of the commonly used nerve blocks and understand their indications and risks. Recognize that sympathetic nerve blocks with local anesthetic may be valuable in some types of cancer-related neuropathic pains. Be aware of the use of prolonged temporary blocks using local anesthetic infusion. Understand the role of neurolytic celiac plexus block in the management of abdominal pain due to cancer of the pancreas and other neoplasms.

C. Be aware of other procedures that may be useful in selected patients with cancer pain, including myofascial trigger point injection, injection of neuroma, use of a cryoprobe for neuroma or nerve block, and use of nitrous oxide for transitory analgesia.

V. Surgical approaches to cancer pain (Arbit 1993)

  A. Recognize that some cancer operations have analgesic consequences, such as repair of bowel obstruction and vertebrectomy for metastatic disease.

  B. Be aware of the common surgical neurolytic procedures, including rhizotomy and cordotomy. Understand the indications and risks for these procedures.

VI. Neurostimulatory approaches to cancer pain (Arbit 1993; Patt 1993)

  A. Recognize that some noninvasive or minimally invasive stimulatory approaches, including counter-irritation, transcutaneous electrical nerve stimulation, and acupuncture, are used empirically for some patients with cancer pain.

  B. Recognize that invasive neurostimulatory approaches, including dorsal column stimulation and deep brain stimulation, are rarely used for cancer pain.

VII. Physiatric approaches to cancer pain (Arbit 1993; Doyle et al. 1993)

  A. Understand that physical therapy can have analgesic consequences, such as prevention of secondary painful myofascial or joint complications in patients with weakened limbs.

  B. Recognize that physical modalities, such as the use of heat or cold, can be used to treat some patients with cancer pain.

VIII. Psychological approaches to cancer pain (Doyle et al. 1993; Patt 1993)

  A. Recognize the range of psychological and psychosocial concerns that may be identified through a comprehensive assessment ,and understand the need to select therapy appropriately.

  B. Understand that psychiatric disorders, most often depression and anxiety disorders, are common among patients with cancer pain, and be aware of the types of problems that should be referred to mental health care providers.

  C. Be aware of the cognitive interventions, such as relaxation training, that may be used to improve pain control or coping with pain, and recognize that some patients with cancer pain can benefit from these techniques.

IX. Special populations with cancer pain

  A. Be aware of the needs of children with cancer pain, including age-appropriate assessment techniques, availability of interventions for procedure-related pain, and adjustments in drug doses.

  B. Be aware of the needs of the elderly with cancer pain, including psychosocial concerns and changes in drug selection and dosing associated with to age-related variation in pharmacokinetics and pharmacodynamics.

C. Be aware of the needs of the substance-abusing population, including the potential for closer monitoring of drug use and the increased likelihood of undertreatment.

D. Be aware of possible cultural differences in the presentation of painful disease, reaction to life-threatening illness, and response to therapies.

REFERENCES

American Society of Clinical Oncology Ad Hoc Committee on Cancer Pain, Cancer pain assessment and treatment guidelines, J. Clin. Oncol., 101 (1992) 1976–1982.

Arbit, E. (Ed.), Management of Cancer-Related Pain. Futura Publishing, Mt. Kisco, NY, 1993.

Cherny, N.I. and Portenoy, R.K., Cancer pain: principles of assessment and syndromes. In: P.D. Wall and R. Melzack (Eds.), Textbook of Pain, 3rd ed., Churchill Livingstone, Edinburgh, 1994a, pp. 787–823.

Cherny, N.I. and Portenoy, R.K., Practical issues in the management of cancer pain. In: P.D. Wall and R. Melzack (Eds.), Textbook of Pain, 3rd ed., Churchill Livingstone, Edinburgh, 1994b, pp. 1437–1467.

Cleeland, C.S., Gonin, R., Hatfield, A.K., Edmonson, J.H., Blum, R.H., Stewart, J.A. and Pandya, K.J., Pain and its treatment in outpatients with metastatic cancer, N. Engl. J. Med., 330 (1994) 592–596.

De Conno F., Caraceni, A., Gamba, A., Mariani, L., Abbattista, A., Brunelli, C., La Mura, A. and Ventafridda V., Pain measurement in cancer patients: a comparison of six methods, Pain, 57 (1994) 161–166.

Doyle, D., Hanks, G.W.C. and MacDonald, N. (Eds.), Oxford Textbook of Palliative Medicine, Oxford University Press, Oxford, 1993.

Eisenberg, E., Berkey, C.S., Carr, D.B., Mosteller, F. and Chalmers, T.C., Efficacy and safety of nonsteroidal antiinflammatory drugs for cancer pain: a meta-analysis, J. Clin. Oncol., 12 (1994) 2756–2765.

Gonzales, G.R., Elliott, K.J., Portenoy, R.K. and Foley, K.M., The impact of a comprehensive evaluation in the management of cancer pain, Pain, 47 (1991) 141–144.

Jacox, A., Carr, D.B. and Payne, R., Management of Cancer Pain, Clinical Practice Guideline No. 9, AHCPR Publication No. 94-0592, U.S. Department of Health and Human Services, Agency for Health Care Policy and Research, Rockville, MD, 1994.

Miser, A.W. and Miser, J.S., The treatment of cancer pain in children, Pediatr. Clin. North Am., 36 (1989) 979–999.

Patt, R.B., Cancer Pain, J.B. Lippincott, Philadelphia, 1993.

Twycross, R., Pain Relief in Advanced Cancer, Churchill Livingstone, Edinburgh, 1994.

World Health Organization, Cancer Pain Relief and Palliative Care, World Health Organization, Geneva, 1992.

Core Curriculum for Professional Education in Pain, edited by H.L. Fields, IASP Press, Seattle, © 1995.

24

Postoperative Pain

I. Be aware of the epidemiology and magnitude of the problem of inadequate pain control after operation, medical procedures, or trauma (including burns) (Bonica 1990; Royal College of Surgeons 1990; Carr et al. 1992; Ogilvy and Smith 1994).

    A. Numbers and prevalence rates of moderate to severe pain in each of these three contexts

    B. Particular burden upon subpopulations: infants and children, the elderly, ethnic minorities or those unable to communicate (Manne et al. 1992; Ekstrom and Ready, in press)

II. Be aware of adverse physiologic effects of acute pain and their modification by anesthetic (regional versus general) and analgesic techniques (Kehlet 1992; Cepeda and Carr, in press).

    A. Metabolic: substrate mobilization, catabolism (particularly protein wasting) mediated largely by hormone secretion (anterior and posterior pituitary, adrenal cortex and medulla, pancreas)

    B. Cardiovascular: hypertension, tachycardia, myocardial ischemia (if coronary artery disease present), lowered fibrillation threshold (neurally and humorally mediated)

    C. Hypercoagulability: risks of thrombotic, embolic disease from immobilization, tissue injury, and hormonal (e.g., epinephrine) actions

    D. Pulmonary compromise due to splinting and intrinsic diaphragmatic muscle impairment (Kavanagh et al. 1994)

    E. Gastrointestinal dysfunction due to pain and pain therapies (especially opioids)

    F. Psychological distress and cognitive dysfunction due to pain and stress hormonal responses (e.g., hypoxia from splinting; hyponatremia due to excessive ADH secretion), helplessness, insomnia, and pain therapies

    G. Predisposition to chronic pain due to central neuronal sensitization, and evidence for and against "preemptive" analgesia to avert such sensitization (Coderre 1993; Dahl and Kehlet 1993; Woolf and Chong 1993; White 1994)

III. Be familiar with the pharmacological properties of the major classes of drugs used for acute pain management, beginning with usual starting doses, frequencies, and comparative (equivalent) doses (Cousins and Phillips 1986; Ready and Edwards 1992; Sinatra et al. 1992; Ferrante and VadeBoncouer 1993).

A. For opioids, know:

1. Major chemical types, receptor selectivity, and agonist features (Chapter 7) of compounds used, to permit rational drug substitution in the presence of adverse reaction or side effects from an agent of one type (e.g., full agonist versus mixed agonist-antagonist or partial agonist; phenylpiperidine versus alkaloid versus peptide) (McQuay 1991)
2. The wide range of durations of actions available through selection of ultra-short (alfentanil, remifentanil) to ultra-long (methadone) acting compounds
3. Common adverse effects (respiratory depression, sedation, constipation, nausea, pruritus, urinary retention), including predisposing patient factors (e.g., prostatism, chronic lung disease) and concurrent drug therapies (e.g., anticholinergics, benzodiazepines), and how to evaluate and treat them
4. The dangers of sudden reversal of perioperative opioid therapy with naloxone
5. Benefits and risks of spinal opioids and evidence for and against the selection of spinal versus systemic routes of opioid administration for specific operative procedures and patients (e.g., comorbidity) (Chrubasik et al. 1993; Cousins 1994)
6. How to approach the opioid treatment of acute pain in the opioid-tolerant patient, whether after deliberate, therapeutic chronic opioid therapy such as for cancer pain, or in the known or suspected substance abuser (Carr et al. 1992; Rapp et al. 1995)

B. For NSAIDs and acetaminophen, know:

1. Alternative routes and dosage forms (e.g., oral, i.v., rectal) (Ballantyne, in press)
2. How to modify doses or withhold NSAIDs in the presence of patient co-morbidity (congestive heart failure, renal disease, ulcer disease, coagulopathy)
3. How to select particular NSAIDs to lessen risk of specific side effects (e.g., nonacetylated compounds for platelet sparing; nabumetone to lessen gastrointestinal blood loss)
4. That there is a "plateau effect" such that dosage increases beyond the recommended range increase the incidence of side effects but do not improve analgesia (Souter et al. 1994)

C. For local anesthetics, know:

1. The anatomy of commonly used nerve blocks (Scott 1989)
2. The major classes of agents, to guide drug substitution in the presence of allergy to one class (i.e., amino-ester versus amide) (Covino 1988)
3. The risks and benefits of addition of epinephrine, or combination analgesia (i.e., local anesthetic plus opioid or NSAIDs)
4. The signs, symptoms, and treatment of systemic local anesthetic toxicity; the risk of toxicity in relation to selection of agent and site of administration; and how to distinguish such toxicity from other common adverse effects of local anesthesia (e.g., hypotension)
5. The indications, risks, benefits and efficacy of local anesthetic application at common peripheral sites (brachial plexus, intercostal nerve, interpleural space) and epidurally

IV. Be able to formulate a comprehensive plan for optimal perioperative pain management based on patient preference, physical and mental status, and available expertise and technology (Carr et al. 1992).

A. Know the indications and contraindications for use of the major drug classes available for acute pain management, and the evidence for their costs and effectiveness when delivered by varied routes (e.g., systemic, spinal) and infusion patterns (e.g., bolus doses, continuous infusion, patient-controlled).

1. Local anesthetics
2. NSAIDS and acetaminophen
3. Opioids
4. Alpha-agonists
5. Other (e.g., tramadol)

B. For patient-controlled analgesia (PCA):

1. Know how to write a "PCA prescription" for opioid administration via systemic (intravenous, subcutaneous) or epidural routes (Ready and Edwards 1992; Ballantyne et al. 1993; White 1994).

   a. Bolus dose
   b. Lockout interval
   c. Basal infusion rate
   d. Dosage limit per time interval (e.g., four or eight hours)

2. Know how to titrate PCA prescription according to clinical need.
3. Be familiar with pros and cons (including expense) of different devices and drugs for systemic PCA used currently (electrical, mechanical) or in late preclinical trials (transbuccal, intranasal, transdermal iontophoretic, inhaled).

C. Be able to manage analgesia during the transitions from "NPO" to oral intake, and from inpatient care through hospital discharge.

D. Be able to select drugs, and adjust doses and delivery techniques, according to the specific needs of the particular patient under treatment (e.g., age, physical status, mental status) and the available resources (e.g., personnel, expertise, budget, monitoring) of the setting in which treatment will be provided.

V. Be familiar with nonpharmacological methods of acute pain control.

A. For transcutaneous electrical nerve stimulation (TENS), know:

1. Evidence for and against its efficacy (compared to sham TENS or no TENS)
2. Techniques of its use (electrode placement and stimulation parameters)

B. For cognitive-behavioral methods (including patient education, relaxation, distraction), know the major approaches, techniques, limitations (e.g., severe pain intensity, or cognitive impairment) and clinical research that favors or opposes their use for acute pain (Carr et al. 1992; Peck 1986).

VI. Know the clinical outcomes (e.g., length and cost of hospitalization, complications due to untreated pain or pain treatments, readmission due to inadequate pain control, patient satisfaction, staff satisfaction) to be evaluated in an organized approach to acute pain management (Kehlet 1992; Miaskowski 1994).

A. Know the types of monitoring (e.g., sedation level, respiratory rate, vital signs) including their frequency of assessment and institutional assignment of responsibility for their performance, that have been recommended by major professional organizations concerned with control of acute pain (Royal College of Surgeons 1990; Ready and Edwards 1992; Ready et al. 1995).

B. Know how to organize an acute pain service that supervises the quality of pain management within an institution, documents institutional performance, ensures the quality of this function, and (if shortfalls arise) recognizes them and prevents their recurrence (Ready et al. 1988; Max et al. 1991; Schug and Haridas 1993; Rawal and Berggren 1994; Ready 1995).

REFERENCES

Ballantyne, J.C., The pharmacology of nonsteroidal anti-inflammatory agents (NSAIDs) for acute postoperative pain. Current Opinion in Anesthesiology, in press.

Ballantyne, J.C., Carr, D.B., Chalmers, T.C., Dear, K.B., Angelillo, I.F. and Mosteller, F., Postoperative patient-controlled meta analyses of initial randomized control trials, J. Clin. Anesth., 5 (1993) 182–193.

Bonica, J.J., Postoperative pain. In: J.J. Bonica (Ed.), The Management of Pain 2nd ed., Lea & Febiger, Philadelphia, 1990, pp. 461–480.

Carr, D.B., Jacox, A.K., Chapman, C.R., et al., Acute Pain Management: Operative or Medical Procedures and Trauma, Clinical Practice Guideline, U.S. Department of Health and Human Services, Public Health Service, Agency for Health Care Policy and Research, Rockville, MD, 1992, AHCPR Pub. No. 92-0032.

Cepeda, M.S. and Carr, D.B., The stress reponse and regional anesthesia. In: D.L. Brown (Ed.), Textbook of Regional Anesthesia and Analgesia, Saunders, Philadelphia, in press.

Chrubasik, J., Chrubasik, S. and Mather, L., Postoperative Epidural Opioids, Springer-Verlag, Berlin, 1993.

Coderre, T.J., Katz, J., Vaccarino, A.L. and Melzack, R., Contribution of central neuroplasticity to pathological pain: review of clinical and experimental evidence, Pain, 52 (1993) 259–285.

Cousins, M.J., The spinal route of analgesia: opioids and future options. In: T.H. Stanley and M.A. Ashburn (Eds.), Anesthesiology and Pain Management, Kluwer Academic Publishers, Dordrecht, 1994, pp.195–226.

Cousins, M.J. and Phillips, G.D. (Eds.), Acute Pain Management, Clinics in Critical Care Medicine, Churchill Livingstone, New York, 1986.

Covino, B.G., Clinical pharmacology of local anesthetic agents. In: M.J. Cousins and P.O. Bridenbaugh (Eds.), Neural Blockade in Clincal Anesthesia and Pain Management, 2nd ed., Lippincott, Philadelphia,1988, pp. 111–144.

Dahl, J.B. and Kehlet, H., The value of pre-emptive analgesia in the treatment of postoperative pain: a critical analysis, Anesth. Analg., 70 (1993) 434–439.

Ekstrom, J.L. and Ready, L.B., Management of acute postoperative pain. In: C.H. McLeskey (Ed.), Geriatric Anesthesiology, Williams & Wilkins, Philadelphia, in press.

Ferrante, F.M. and VadeBoncouer, T.R. (Eds.), Postoperative Pain Management, Churchill Livingstone, New York, 1993, pp. 79–106.

Kavanagh, B.P., Katz, J. and Sandler, A.N., Pain control following thoracic surgery: a review of the current status, Anesthesiology, 81 (1994) 737–759.

Kehlet, H., General vs regional anesthesia, In: M.R. Rogers, J.H. Tinker, B.G. Covino and D.E. Longnecker (Eds.), Principles and Practice of Anesthesiology, Mosby-Year Book, London, 1992.

Kehlet, H., Postoperative pain relief: a look from the other side, Reg. Anesth., 19 (1994) 369–377.

Manne, S.L., Jacobsen, P.B. and Redd, W.H., Assessment of acute pediatric pain: do child self-report, parent ratings and nurse ratings measure the same phenomenon? Pain, 48 (1992) 45–52.

Max, M.B., Donovan, M., Portenoy, R.K., et al., American Pain Society quality assurance standards for relief of acute pain and cancer pain. In: M.R. Bond, J.E. Charlton and C.J. Woolf (Eds.), Proceedings of the VIth World Congress on Pain, Vol. 4, Elsevier, Amsterdam, 1991, pp. 185–189.

McQuay, H.J., Opioid clinical pharmacology and routes of administration. In: J.C.D. Wells and C.J. Woolf (Eds.), Br. Med. Bull., 81 (1991) 737–759.

Miaskowski, C., Pain management: quality assurance and changing practice. In: G.F. Gebhart, D.L. Hammond and T.S. Jensen (Eds.), Proceedings of the 7th World Congress on Pain, Progress in Pain Research and Management, Vol. 2, IASP Press, Seattle, 1994, pp. 75–96.

Ogilvy, A.J. and Smith, G., Postoperative pain. In: W.S. Nimmo, D.J. Rowbotham and G. Smith (Eds.), Anaesthesia (2nd ed.), Blackwell Scientific Publications, Oxford, 1994, pp. 1570–1601.

Peck, C.L., Psychological factors in acute pain management. In: M.J. Cousins and G.D. Phillips (Eds.), Acute Pain Management, Clinics in Critical Care Medicine, Churchill Livingstone, New York, 1986, pp. 251–274.

Rapp, S.E., Ready, L.B. and Nessly, M.L., Acute pain management in patients with prior opioid consumption: a case-controlled retrospective study, Pain, 61 (1995) 195–201.

Rawal, N. and Berggren, L., Organization of acute pain services: a low-cost model, Pain, 57 (1994) 117–123.

Ready, L.B., How many acute pain services are there in the United States and who is managing patient-controlled analgesia? Anesthesiology, 82 (1995) 322.

Ready, L.B. and Edwards, W.T. (Eds.), Management of Acute Pain: A Practical Guide, IASP Press, Seattle, 1992.

Ready, L.B., Ashburn, M., Caplan, R.A., et al., Practice guidelines for acute pain management in the perioperative setting, Anesthesiology, 82 (1995) 1071–1081.

Ready, L.B., Oden, R., Chadwick, H.S., Benedetti, C., Rooke, G.A., Caplan, R. and Wild, L.M., Development of an anesthesiology-based postoperative pain service, Anesthesiology, 68 (1988) 100–106.

Royal College of Surgeons of England and the College of Anesthetists, Report of the Working Party on Pain after Surgery, Royal College of Surgeons, London, 1990.

Schug, S.A. and Haridas, R.P., Development and organizational structure of an acute pain service in a major teaching hospital. Aust. N. Z. J. Surg., 63 (1993) 8–13.

Scott, D.B., Techniques of Regional Anaesthesia, Appleton and Lange, Norwalk, 1989.

Sinatra, R.S., Hord, A.H., Ginsberg, B. and Preble, L.M. (Eds.), Acute Pain: Mechanisms and Management, Mosby–Year Book, St. Louis, 1992.

Souter, A.J., Fredman, B. and White, P.F., Controversies in the perioperative use of antiinflammatory drugs. Anesth. Analg., 79 (1994) 1178–1190.

White, P.F., Patient controlled analgesia (Part 1 & Part 2). In: T.H. Stanley and M.A. Ashburn (Eds.), Anesthesiology and Pain Management, Kluwer Academic Publishers, Dordrecht, 1994, pp. 117–142.

Woolf, C.J. and Chong, M-S., Preemptive analgesia - treating postoperative pain by preventing the establishment of central sensitization, Anesth. Analg., 77 (1993) 362–379.

Yaksh, T.L. and Abram, S.E., Preemptive analgesia: a popular misnomer, but a clinically relevant truth? APS Journal, 2 (1993) 116–121.

Core Curriculum for Professional Education in Pain, edited by H.L. Fields, IASP Press, Seattle, © 1995.

25

Compensation, Disability Assessment, Pain in the Workplace

I. Understand the difference between disease, impairment, disability, and functional capacity. Recognize that while pain is a complex phenomenon, impairments are medically determinable and measurable objectively, while disability is a "task-specific" limitation of function (Osterweis et al. 1987; Chapman and Brena 1989; American Medical Association 1992; Sanders et al. 1995; Vasudevan 1992; Vasudevan and Monsein 1992).

II. Recognize that in many patients with chronic pain, it may be difficult to make a diagnosis, especially if soft tissue problems are overlooked (American Medical Association 1992).

III. Be aware that chronic pain can produce impairment due to sensory input that affects the musculoskeletal system through limiting or altering patterns of movement, strength, and endurance; the central nervous system producing cognitive and emotional disturbances (Chapman and Brena 1989; Mendelson 1994).

IV. Understand that there are several approaches for evaluating disability and that a systematic approach to understanding different disability systems and the preparation of a report can be helpful to both the patient and the physician (Vasudevan 1992).

V. Know that despite minimal objective evidence of impairment, patients who have chronic pain may have severe functional deficits and perceive that they cannot carry out their normal functions as long as they have pain. (Pettingill 1979; Follick et al. 1985; Naliboff 1985; Riley et al. 1988).

VI. Recognize that there is conflicting evidence regarding compensation and litigation issues and consequences for the evaluation and treatment of chronic pain patients.

A. There is evidence that compensation patients report more functional and vocational dysfunction related to their pain syndromes than do noncompensation patients (Leavitt et al. 1982; Tart et al. 1988) and that patients receiving compensation respond less favorably to a variety of treatments than do patients who are not receiving compensation (Mendelson 1982, 1986; Labbe et al. 1988; Weighill and Burglass 1989; Fishbain 1994). Other studies, however, indicate that the poor short-term outcome in patients with compensation is more closely related to unemployment (Dworkin 1985).

B. Be aware of evidence that litigation *per se* plays at most a minor role in influencing treatment outcome in chronic pain (Solomon and Tunks 1991).

C. Recognize that although "compensation patients" with physical findings have been psychiatrically labeled, (Ford 1977-78; Sim 1982; Weighill 1983), the labels are not recognized in the DSM-IV nomenclature (American Psychiatric Association 1994).

VII.   Recognize that, for injured workers, returning to work is complicated by a variety of factors including employer attitudes, self-doubt following long periods of unemployment, fear of reinjury, fear of not being able to manage pain at the workplace, and fear of not being able to reinstate disability in case of failure (Chapman and Brena 1989).

VIII. Be aware that data comparing the disability period of employees with back injuries suffered on duty, versus those sustained off duty, indicate a longer period of disability for injuries sustained at work; the difference is statistically significant even when cases are matched for gender and activity (Sander and Meyers 1986).

IX.   Understand that the objective physical impairment in patients with chronic pain accounts for less than half of the total disability. Other psychological and behavioral factors, especially depression and increased bodily awareness, family structure and income, regional unemployment rates, ability of the worker to control his/her work pace and work task, cultural values, and education level are important determinants of return to work (Waddell 1984; Chapman and Brena 1989).

X.   Be aware that patients with "nonorganic physical findings" can be disabled due to their pain (Miller 1961; Dworkin et al. 1985; Tarsh and Royston 1985) and may benefit from use of clinical practice guidelines that have been proposed for treating patients with chronic nonmalignant pain syndrome (Sanders et al. 1995).

XI.   Be aware that the definition of malingering includes a *conscious* desire to deceive for potential secondary gain (Gorman 1982; Stevens 1986; American Psychiatric Association 1994).

XII.   Be aware of data that malingering occurs in 5% or fewer of patients with low back pain (Austerities et al. 1987; Chapman and Brena 1989). Know that neither the DSM-IV nor the ICD-10 include malingering as a diagnosis (Mendelson and Mendelson 1993; World Health Organization 1992).

XIII. Understand the concept of secondary gain (Martin 1974; Merskey 1988; Fishbain 1994).

XIV.   Understand that disability is both task specific and role specific.

XV.   Understand the role of health professionals in the assessment of disability (Vasudevan 1992; Vasudevan and Monsein 1992).

REFERENCES

American Medical Association, Guides to the Evaluation of Permanent Impairment, 4th ed., American Medical Association, Chicago, 1992.

American Psychiatric Association staff, Diagnostic and Statistical Manual of Mental Disorders, DSM-IV, American Psychiatric Association, Washington, D.C., 1994.

Chapman, S.L. and Brena, S.F., Pain and litigation. In: P.D. Wall and R. Melzack (Eds.), Textbook of Pain, Churchill Livingstone, Edinburgh, 1989.

Dworkin, R.H., Handlin, D.S., Richlin, D.M., Brand, L. and Vannucci, C., Unraveling the effects of compensation, litigation, and employment on treatment response in chronic pain, Pain, 23 (1985) 49–59.

Fishbain, D.A., Goldberg, M., Labbe, E., Steele, R. and Rosomoff, H., Compensation and non compensation chronic pain patients compared for DSM-III operational diagnoses, Pain, 32 (1988) 197–206.

Fishbain, D.A., Secondary Gain Concept: definition problems and its abuse in medical practice, APS Journal, 3 (1994) 264–273.

Follick, M.J., Smith, T.W. and Ahern, D.K., The Sickness Impact Profile: a global measure of disability in chronic low back pain, Pain, 21 (1985) 67–76.

Ford, C.V., A type of disability neurosis: the Humpty Dumpty Syndrome, Intl. J. Psychiatry Med., 8 (1977–78) 285–294.

Gorman, W.F., Defining malingering, J. Forensic Sci., 27 (1982) 401–407.

Labbe, E.E., Fishbain, D., Goldberg, M., Steele-Rosomoff, R. and Rosomoff, H.L., Compensation and non-compensation pain patients: responses to the Millon Behavioral Health Inventory, Pain Manage., 1 (1988) 133–139.

Leavitt, F., Garron, D.C., McNeill, T.W. and Whistler, W.W., Organic status, psychological disturbance, and pain report characteristics in low-back-pain patients on compensation, Spine, 7 (1982) 398–402.

Martin, R.D., Secondary gain, everybody's rationalization, J. Occup. Med., 16 (1974) 800–801.

Mendelson, G., Not "cured by a verdict." Effect of legal settlement on compensation claimants, Med. J. Aust., 2 (1982) 132–134.

Mendelson, G., Chronic pain and compensation: a review, J. Pain Symptom Manage., 1 (1986) 135–144.

Mendelson, G., Chronic pain and compensation issues. In: P.D. Wall and R. Melzack (Eds.) Textbook of Pain, 3rd ed., Churchill-Livingstone, Edinburgh, 1994, pp. 1387–1400.

Mendelson, G. and Mendelson, D., Legal and psychiatric aspects of malingering, Journal of Law and Medicine, 1 (1993) 23–34.

Merskey, H., Regional pain is rarely hysterical, Arch. Neurol., 45 (1988) 915–918.

Miller, H., Accident neurosis, Brit. Med. J., 1 (1961) 919–925.

Naliboff, B.D., Cohen, M.J., Swanson, G.A., Bonebakker, A.D. and McArthur, D.L., Comprehensive assessment of chronic low back pain patients and controls: physical abilities, level of activity, psychological adjustment and pain perception, Pain, 23 (1985) 121–134.

Osterweis, M., Kleinman, A. and Mechanic, D. (Eds.), Pain and Disability: Clinical, Behavioral, and Public Policy Perspectives, National Academy Press, Washington DC, 1987.

Pettingill, B.F., Physicians' estimates of disability vs. patients' reports of pain, Psychosomatics, 20 (1979) 827–830.

Riley, J.F., Ahern, D.K. and Follick, M.J., Chronic low back pain and functional impairment: assessing beliefs about their relationship, Arch. Phys. Med. Rehabil., 69 (1988) 579–582.

Rosomoff, H.L., Fishbain, D.A., Goldberg, M., Santana, R. and Steele-Rosomoff, R., Physical findings in patients with chronic intractable benign pain of the neck and/or back, Pain, 37 (1989) 279–287.

Sander, R.A. and Meyers, J.E., The relationship of disability to compensation states in railroad workers, Spine, 11 (2) (1986) 14.

Sanders, S.H., Rucker, K.S., Anderson, K.D., Harden, R.N., Jackson, K.W., Vincente, P.J. and Gallagher, R.M., Clinical practice guidelines for chronic nonmalignant pain syndrome patients, Journal of Back and Musculoskeletal Rehabilitation, 5 (1995) 115–120.

Sim, M., The management of hysteria. In: A. Roy (Ed.), Hysteria, John Wiley & Sons, New York, 1982, pp. 266–267.

Solomon, P. and Tunks, E., The role of litigation in predicting disability outcomes in chronic pain patients, Clin. J. Pain, 7 (1991) 300–304.

Stevens, H., Is it organic or is it functional, is it hysteria or malingering? Psychiatric Clin. N. Amer., 9 (1986) 241–255.

Stinnett, J.L., The functional somatic symptom, Psychiatric Clin. N. Amer., 10 (1987) 19–33.

Tait, R.C., Margolis, R.B., Krause, S.J. and Liebowitz, E., Compensation status and symptoms reported by patients with chronic pain, Arch. Phys. Med. Rehab., 69 (1988) 1027–1029.

Tarsh, M.J. and Royston, C., A follow-up study of accident neurosis, Br. J. Psychiatry, 146 (1985) 18–25.

Vasudevan, S.V., Impairment, disability, and functional capacity assessment. In: Handbook of Pain Assessment, D.C. Turk and R. Melzack (Eds.), Guilford Press, New York, 1992.

Vasudevan, S.V. and Monsein, M., Evaluation of function and disability in the patient with chronic pain. In: Practical Management of Pain, 2nd ed., Mosby–Year Book, St. Louis, 1992.

Waddell, G., Main, C.J., Morris, E.W., Di Paola, M. and Gray, I.C.M., Chronic low back pain, psychological distress and illness behavior, Spine, 9 (2) (1984) 209–213.

Weighill, V.E., Compensation neurosis: a review of the literature, J. Psychosom. Res., 27 (1983) 97–104.

Weighill, V.E. and Buglass, D., An updated review of compensation neurosis, Pain Management, 2 (1989) 100–105.

World Health Organization, The ICD-10 Classification of Mental and Behavioral Disorders—Clinical description and diagnostic guidelines, World Health Organization, Geneva, 1992.

Core Curriculum for Professional Education in Pain, edited by H.L. Fields, IASP Press, Seattle, © 1995.

26

Orofacial Pain, Including Temporomandibular Disorders

I. Anatomical, physiological, and psychological aspects of orofacial pain (Dubner et al. 1978; Sessle 1987; Dworkin and LeResche 1992; Zarb et al. 1994; Fricton and Dubner 1995; Sessle et al. 1995)

   A. Know the peripheral nerve distribution of the major trigeminal nerve trunks and other nerves of the head and mouth, the anatomic relations of the structures they innervate, and their primary central connections.

   B. Be aware of the commonalties between the trigeminal system and the spinal and lemniscal systems that make current concepts of nociceptive transmission and its control applicable to the trigeminal system.

   C. Similarly, be aware of features that distinguish these systems, e.g., in the trigeminal system, the proportion of myelinated to unmyelinated fibers and the properties of some of these fibers are different from those in spinal nerves; the occurrence of sites (e.g., tooth pulp, cornea) in the orofacial region that are predominantly or exclusively innervated by nociceptive afferents; the bilateral and disproportionately large representation of the orofacial region in higher levels of the somatosensory system; the nuclear and subnuclear organization of the trigeminal brainstem complex; the exquisite sensibility of orofacial tissues.

   D. Be aware of the important psychological meaning of the orofacial area and of the role of psychological and psychosocial factors in orofacial pain conditions.

II. Diagnosis of orofacial pain (Fricton et al. 1988; Raskin 1988; Fromm and Sessle 1991; Attanasio and Mohl 1992; Dworkin and LeResche 1992; McNeil et al. 1993; Loeser 1994; Sharav 1994; Zarb et al. 1994; Fricton and Dubner 1995; Okeson 1995; Sessle et al. 1995)

   A. Be aware of the major diagnostic features and possible etiological, epidemiological, and pathophysiological aspects of pain associated with:

      1. Specific sites: tooth (e.g., pulpitis, periapical periodontitis), temporomandibular joint, muscle, mucosa, sinus, bone, salivary glands
      2. Orofacial pain conditions and syndromes: neuropathic pain (e.g., trigeminal and glossopharyngeal neuralgia, postherpetic neuralgia, deafferentation pain), temporomandibular disorders (including myofascial pain and internal derangements of the temporomandibular joint), vascular-type pain (e.g., cluster headache, migraine, carotidynia), burning mouth, atypical odontalgia, atypical facial pain

   B. Be aware that there are objective and validated tests and procedures used for differential diagnosis of many of the above but that some diagnostic approaches still lack reliability, validity, specificity, or selectivity (Fricton et al. 1988; Sharav 1994; Zarb et al. 1994; Okeson 1995; Sessle et al. 1995). Some of the commonly used tests and procedures include tooth pulp vitality and tooth percussion tests, muscle palpation tests, and other physical exams; behavioral and psychosocial assessments; radiographs and other imaging techniques; microbiological and serological tests; and nerve blocks.

    C. Know the common orofacial patterns of pain referral (Fricton et al. 1988; Sharav 1994; Okeson 1995). Also be aware that orofacial pain may sometimes be referred from remote sites (e.g., earache, cardiac pain, intracranial lesions).

III.   Treatment of orofacial pain (Fricton et al. 1988; Fromm and Sessle 1991; Attanasio and Mohl 1992; McNeil et al. 1993; Loeser 1994; Zarb et al. 1994; Fricton and Dubner 1995; Okeson 1995; Sessle et al. 1995)

    A. Be familiar with the treatments advocated for the different types of orofacial pain noted in section II above. Some of the commonly used therapeutic approaches include pharmacological agents, surgery, physical medicine, and multidisciplinary approaches.

    B. Be aware of the indications and contraindications of these therapeutic approaches.

REFERENCES

Attanasio, R. and Mohl, N., Educational guidelines of temporomandibular disorders, J. Craniomandib. Disord. Facial Oral Pain, 6 (1992) 123–134.

Dworkin, S.F. and LeResche, L., Research diagnostic criteria for temporomandibular disorders: review, criteria, examinations and specifications, critique, J. Craniomandib. Disord. Facial Oral Pain, 6 (1992) 301–355.

Dubner, R., Sessle, B.J. and Storey, A.T., The Neural Basis of Oral and Facial Function, Plenum, New York, 1978.

Fricton, J. and Dubner, R., Advances in Temporomandibular Disorders and Orofacial Pain, Raven Press, New York, 1995.

Fricton, J.R., Kroening, R.J. and Hathaway, K.M., TMJ and Craniofacial Pain: Diagnosis and Management, Ishiyaku Euro America, St. Louis, 1988.

Fromm, G.H. and Sessle, B.J., Trigeminal Neuralgia: Current Concepts Regarding Pathogenesis and Treatment, Butterworths, Stoneham, 1991.

Loeser, J.D., Tic douloureux and atypical face pain. In: P.D. Wall and R. Melzack (Eds.), Textbook of Pain, 3rd ed., Churchill Livingstone, Edinburgh, 1994, pp. 699–710.

McNeil, C., et al., Temporomandibular Disorders: Guidelines for Evaluation, Diagnosis, and Management (American Academy of Orofacial Pain), 2nd ed., Quintessence, Chicago, 1993.

Okeson, J.P., Bell's Orofacial Pains, 5th ed., Quintessence, Chicago, 1995.

Raskin, N.H., Facial pain. In: Headache, 2nd ed., Churchill Livingstone, New York, 1988, pp. 333–373.

Sessle, B.J., The neurobiology of facial and dental pain: present knowledge, future directions, J. Dent. Res., 66 (1987) 962–981.

Sessle, B.J., Bryant, P.S. and Dionne, R.A., Temporomandibular Disorders and Related Pain Conditions, IASP Press, Seattle, 1995.

Sharav, Y., Orofacial pain. In: P.D. Wall and R. Melzack (Eds.), Textbook of Pain, 3rd ed., Churchill Livingstone, Edinburgh, 1994, pp. 563–582.

Zarb, G.A., Carlsson, G.E., Sessle, B.J. and Mohl, N.D., Temporomandibular Joint and Masticatory Muscle Disorders, Munksgaard, Copenhagen, 1994.

Core Curriculum for Professional Education in Pain, edited by H.L. Fields, IASP Press, Seattle, © 1995.

27

Animal Models of Pain
and Ethics of Animal Experimentation

I. Animal Models of Pain (Vonvoigtlander 1982; Wood 1984; Dubner 1987; Dubner 1994)

A. Know criteria that define useful and ethical animal models of pain.

B. Know the characteristics and uses of the following animal models of pain:

1. Tail or paw withdrawal to thermal stimulation (e.g., tail-flick test)
2. Hot-plate test
3. Tooth pulp stimulation
4. Paw or intra-articular injections of yeast, formalin, carageenan, adjuvant, etc.
5. Intraperitoneal injections of irritant solutions
6. Hollow organ distention
7. Constriction or compression of peripheral or spinal nerves or roots
8. Partial or complete transection of peripheral or spinal nerves or roots

C. Know which tests measure changes in reflexes and which measure changes in behavior; know the central nervous system (CNS) level of organization of the response and the extent to which sensory and motor components contribute to interpretation of results.

D. Know which tests model tonic pain, phasic pain, visceral pain, neuropathic pain, inflammation, or other pain conditions (Mason et al. 1985; Bennett and Xie 1988; Ness and Gebhart 1988).

E. Know the extent to which the model and pathology (if present) replicate a pain condition in humans, and the extent to which treatments predict application to humans. Know whether and why or why not the model conforms to ethical guidelines for animal use (see below).

II. Ethics of animal experimentation (IASP 1983; Caplan 1986; Dubner 1987; Fox and Mickley 1986, 1987)

A. Understand moral and ethical issues and arguments associated with the use of nonhuman animals for experimentation.

B. Understand and subscribe to the need to justify the use of animals to both the scientific and nonscientific communities.

C. Know how to design experiments that minimize the numbers of animals used (know how to determine the required number), that maximize statistical inferences, and that maximize the recording of variables relevant to the assessment of pain experienced by the animals.

D. Know how to employ a nociceptive stimulus or condition (e.g., inflammation) that is minimal in intensity and duration (tested on the investigator when possible) so as to shorten the duration of an experiment consistent with the attainment of justifiable, ethical research objectives.

E. Know reasons why unanesthetized animals should not be exposed to nociceptive stimuli from which they cannot escape, avoid, or terminate, and why pharmacologically paralyzed animals also should be anesthetized or rendered neurosurgically insensate.

F. Know the International Association for the Study of Pain guidelines establishing ethical standards for animal experimentation (IASP 1983).

REFERENCES

Bennett, G.J. and Xie, Y.-K., A peripheral mononeuropathy in rat that produces disorders of pain sensation like those seen in man, Pain, 33 (1988) 87–108.

Caplan, A., Moral community and the responsibility of scientists, Acta. Physiol. Scand. Suppl., 128 (554) (1986) 78–90.

Committee on Pain and Distress in Laboratory Animals, Institute of Laboratory Animal Resources, Commission on Life Sciences, National Research Council, Recognition and Alleviation of Pain and Distress in Laboratory Animals, National Academy Press, Washington, D.C., 1992.

Dubner, R., Research on pain mechanisms in animals, J. Am.Vet. Med. Assoc., 191 (1987) 1273–1276.

Dubner, R., Methods of assessing pain in animals. In: P.D. Wall and R. Melzack (Eds.), Textbook of Pain, Churchill Livingstone, Edinburgh, 1994, pp. 293–302.

Fox, M.W. and Mickley, L.D. (Eds.), Advances in Animal Welfare Science, Martinus Nijhoff Publishers, Boston, 1986 and 1987. (This is a series with many useful chapters relating to ethics and laboratory animal welfare.)

International Association for the Study of Pain, Ethical guidelines for investigations of experimental pain in conscious animals, Pain, 16 (1983) 109–110.

Mason, P., Strassman, A. and Maciewicz, R., Is the jaw-opening reflex a valid model of pain? Brain Res. Rev., 10 (1985) 137–146.

Ness, T.J. and Gebhart, G.F., Colorectal distension as a noxious visceral stimulus: physiologic and pharmacologic characterization of pseudaffective reflexes in the rat, Brain Res., 450 (1988) 153–169.

Vonvoigtlander, P.F., Pharmacological alteration of pain: the discovery and evaluation of analgetics in animals. In: D. Lednicer (Ed.), Central Analgetics, John Wiley & Sons, New York, 1982, pp. 51–79.

Wood, P.L., Animal models in analgesic testing. In: M. Kuhar and G. Pasternak (Eds.), Analgesics: Neurochemical, Behavioral and Clinical Perspectives, Raven Press, New York, 1984, pp. 175–194.

Core Curriculum for Professional Education in Pain, edited by H.L. Fields, IASP Press, Seattle, © 1995.

28

Pain in Children

I. Understand the multidimensional nature of children's pain experiences.

   A. Know about the developmental biology of pain in infants.

   B. Know about the developmental psychology of pain in infants and children.

   C. Know the factors (situational, behavioral, emotional, and familial) that modify children's pain perceptions and pain behaviors.

   D. Know how to differentiate the myths about children's pain experiences (e.g., neonates don't require analgesics) from the reality demonstrated in empirical studies.

   E. Know about the role of parents in pain measurement and treatment in children.

   F. Be aware of differences in the spectrum of pain experienced by children and adults.

II. Be aware of methods of pain measurement and assessment in children.

   A. Know that pain assessment and pain management are inextricably linked.

   B. Know the principal behavioral and physiological measures for assessing distress in infants and children.

   C. Know the limitations for inferring pain from physiological and behavioral distress responses.

   D. Know the principal self-report methods for assessing pain in children (e.g., scales and interviews).

   E. Know how to select measures for clinical use and ensure that children can use them.

   F. Know that routine measurement and recording of pain is an important aspect of pain management of children in hospitals.

   G. Know that comprehensive pain assessment requires a thorough assessment of the pain in relation to the child and the factors (environmental and internal) that modify the pain, not only identification of the source of noxious stimulation.

   H. Know that structured interviews combined with quantitative pain scales (e.g., visual analog scales) provide the best measures for assessing acute, recurrent, and chronic pain.

III.   Pharmacological interventions for alleviating children's pain

    A.   Know that controlling children's pain requires an integrated approach because many factors are responsible, no matter how seemingly clear-cut the cause.

    B.   Ensure that appropriate health professionals assume responsibility for evaluating pain and for prescribing and administering medications.

    C.   Know about management of physical drug dependence. Know that producing addiction is not a problem in pain management in children.

    D.   Know the guidelines for analgesia administration in infants, children, and adolescents. Be aware that anesthetics are safe and humane for neonates but should be administered in an institution capable of managing neonates.

    E.   Know that you are not treating pain as an entity distinct from the child, but that you are treating a child with pain.

    F.   Know the neonatal and child pharmacokinetics and pharmacodynamics of the major opioid and nonopioid analgesics used with neonates and children.

    G.   Know that a sense of control is important to children and that analgesic administration should involve their active participation (when possible) to minimize pain.

    H.   Know about advisability of using methods of drug administration that are well accepted by children and that prevent reoccurrence of pain.

    I.   Know that adequate analgesic medications, administered at regular dosing intervals, should be complemented by practical cognitive-behavioral methods to ensure optimal pain relief.

    J.   Regularly document a child's pain pre- and posttreatment to evaluate analgesic efficacy.

IV.   Nonpharmacological methods for alleviating children's pain

    A.   Know behavioral interventions and their applications, such as relaxation and biofeedback, and exercise.

    B.   Know primary cognitive methods and their applications, such as distraction, attention, hypnosis, and guided imagery.

    C.   Know why multistrategy programs for reducing pain may be the most appropriate treatment for pediatric pain problems, such as treatment-induced pain, recurrent pain syndromes, and chronic pain.

    D.   Know how to select and integrate methods to optimally reduce a child's pain.

V.   Acute pain

    A.   Know the management of the common acute pains during childhood, e.g., postoperative pain, procedural pain, burns, and medical diseases.

B. Be aware of how to monitor children requiring opioids and understand the importance of respiratory rate, sedation scores, pulse oximetry, and the effects of opioids on pulse rate and blood pressure.

C. Be aware of the indications for major regional blockade, the advantages and disadvantages, and management protocols. Be aware of the place of simple local anesthetic procedures (e.g., wound infiltration, topical creams) in the management of pediatric pain.

D. Be aware of the common side effects of analgesic therapy and be able to achieve a suitable balance between pain relief and side effects.

E. Appreciate the advantages and disadvantages of anxiolytic and amnesic agents such as midazolam for treatment of acute pain.

F. Appreciate the benefits of combining analgesic techniques for better effect.

G. Know the dangers and limitations of intravenous sedation and appreciate the need for monitoring and appropriate staff training.

VI. Recurrent pain

A. Know that many otherwise psychologically and physically healthy children suffer from recurrent pains (e.g., headache, abdominal pain, limb pain).

B. Know about the causes and treatments of recurrent headache, abdominal pain, limb pain, and chest pain.

C. Know that children with recurrent pain are at risk for developing "learned or conditioned" pain triggers, as they usually are searching for environmental causes for the variable painful episodes.

D. Know that children and parents require an explicit diagnosis and information about the causative and contributing factors.

VII. Chronic or persistent pain

A. Know the primary situational, emotional, and behavioral factors that affect a child's chronic or persistent pain, as a function of age.

B. Know about the childhood diseases that are associated with chronic or persistent pain and the best approaches to pain management (e.g., arthritis, sympathetically maintained pain, cancer, sickle cell disease).

C. Know that the management of chronic pain in children necessitates a multidisciplinary approach for optimal management, because the pain is often due to multiple sources affecting both peripheral and central mechanisms, and is modified by many situational, emotional, and behavioral factors.

REFERENCES

Anand, K.J.S. and McGrath, P.J., Pain in Neonates, Elsevier, Amsterdam, 1993.

Barr, R.G., Pain experience in children: developmental and clinical characteristics. In: P.D. Wall and R. Melzack (Eds.), Textbook of Pain, 3rd ed., Churchill Livingstone, London, 1994, pp. 739–768.

Berde, C.B., Lehn, B.M., Yee, J.D., Sethna, N.F. and Russo, D., Patient-controlled analgesia in children and adolescents: a randomized, prospective comparison with intramuscular administration of morphine for postoperative analgesia, J. Pediatr., 118 (1991) 460–466.

Fitzgerald, M., Neurobiology of fetal and neonatal pain. In: P.D. Wall and R. Melzack (Eds.), Textbook of Pain, 3rd ed., Churchill Livingstone, London, 1994, pp. 153–164.

Gaukroger, P.B., Pain management consultation in pediatric patients. In: R.R. Kirby and N. Gravenstein (Eds.), Clinical Anesthesia Practice, W.B. Saunders, Philadelphia, 1994, pp. 261–275.

Karl, H.W., Midazolam sedation for pediatric patients, Curr. Opin. Anesthesiol., 6 (1993) 509–514.

Maunuksela, E.L., Nonsteroidal anti-inflammatory drugs in pediatric pain management. In: N.L. Schechter, C.B. Berde and M. Yaster (Eds.), Pain in Infants, Children, and Adolescents, Williams & Wilkins, Baltimore, 1993, pp. 135–144.

McCaffery, M. and Beebe, A., Pain: Clinical Manual for Nursing Practice, C.V. Mosby, St. Louis, 1989.

McGrath, P.A., Pain in Children: Nature, Assessment and Treatment, Guilford Press, New York, 1990.

McGrath, P.J. and Unruh, A., Pain in Children and Adolescents, Elsevier Science Publishers, Amsterdam, 1987.

Miser, A.W., Management of pain associated with childhood cancer. In: N.L. Schechter, C.B. Berde and M. Yaster (Eds.), Pain in Infants, Children, and Adolescents, Williams & Wilkins, Baltimore, 1993, pp. 411–424.

Olkola, K.T., Hamunen, K. and Maunuksela, E.-L., Clinical Pharmacokinetics and pharmacodynamics of opioid analgesics in infants and children, Clin. Pharmacokinet., 28 (1995) 385–404.

Pichard-Leandri, E. and Gauvain-Piquard, A., La Douleur Dhez L'enfant, Medsi/McGraw-Hill, Paris, 1989.

Schechter, N.L. (Ed.), Acute pain in children, Pediatr. Clin. North Am., 36 (1989) 781–1047.

Schechter, N.L., Berde, C.B. and Yaster, M. (Eds.), Pain in Infants, Children, and Adolescents, Williams & Wilkins, Baltimore, 1993.

Shapiro, B.S., Schechter, N.L. and Ohene-Frempong, K., Conference Proceedings, Sickle Cell Disease Related Pain: Asessment and Management. In: The Genetic Resource, Special Issue, New England Regional Genetics Group (NERGG), Mt. Desert, ME, 1994, pp. 1-53.

Walker, L.S. and Greene, J.W., Children with recurrent abdominal pain and their parents: more somatic complaints, anxiety, and depression than other patient families? J. Pediatr. Psychol., 14 (1989) 231-243.

Core Curriculum for Professional Education in Pain, edited by H.L. Fields, IASP Press, Seattle, © 1995.

29

Ethical Standards in Pain Management and Research

I. General concepts

A. Philosophical concepts

1. Understand common confusions about the concepts of subjective experience of pain and objective assessment of pain, and ways these confusions have contributed to problems in research and practice (Schrag 1982; Scarry 1985; Vrancken 1989; Rollin 1990; Max 1992; Cunningham 1993; Cassell 1995).

2. Understand the distinction between the concepts of pain and suffering, and ways this distinction may or may not give scientific and moral status to the emotional component of pain (Schrag 1982; Stein 1985; Loewy 1991; Roy 1992; Shapiro 1995).

3. Be aware of ways in which scientific and clinical attention to individual and group differences in the intensity and meaning of pain may conflict with the scientific ideal of predictable, universal causes and markers of pain (Krystal 1971; Vrancken 1989; Acute Pain Management Guideline Panel 1992a; Acute Pain Management Guideline Panel 1992b; Anderson and Anderson 1994; Somerville 1994; Cassell 1995).

B. Ethical obligations

1. Be aware that while international groups (including IASP) have accepted the importance of respecting individual cultures, they have also insisted upon basic human rights and responsibilities, and the consequent need for change of current practices (Foley 1994; Miaskowski 1994; Somerville 1994; CIOMS 1995).

2. Understand the moral claim that witnesses to patients' suffering of unnecessary pain have a moral responsibility to those patients, even if the witnesses are not clinically responsible for the patients (Loewy 1991; Hilberg 1992; Institute of Medicine 1994). Understand the potential moral difficulties associated with professionals' development of emotional distance from patients in pain (Stein 1985; Geach 1987; Gadow 1989; Shapiro and Ferrell 1992; Cunningham 1993; Somerville 1994; Cassell 1995; Shapiro 1995).

3. Understand that moderate to excruciating pain can be physically and psychologically harmful; therefore, preventing or alleviating such pain is not merely a matter of charity or doing good (beneficence), but also duty or preventing harm (nonmaleficence) (Bonica 1953; Melzack 1988; Loewy 1991; Acute Pain Management Guideline Panel 1992b; Carr 1993; Walco et al. 1994).

4. Be aware that patients in pain may be at great risk for injury to their dignity, as well as to their autonomy; patients whose pain has been ignored, especially iatrogenic pain, may experience their pain in the same way as do victims of torture (Krystal 1971; Scarry 1985; Gadow 1989;

Randall and Lutz 1991; Somerville 1994; Cowart 1995). International moral rules proscribe torture or other degrading treatment (U.N. Commission on Human Rights 1948).

5. Understand the principle of justice as it may apply to all individuals and groups of patients in areas of pain prevention, assessment, and treatment (Foley 1994). Defending current practice merely by pointing to historical or current standard practice may be a form of false justice (Mount 1990; Cunningham 1993; Walco et al. 1994; International Association for the Study of Pain, in press).

II. Clinical Care

A. Professional power and responsibility

1. Be aware of the scope of power professionals have over patients and families, including physical, bureaucratic, psychological, informational, political, and economic. Understand the moral sensitivity required to use of each these forms of power in a supportive manner, rather than an indifferent or abusive one (Scarry 1985; Gadow 1989; Brody 1992; Roy 1992; Shapiro and Ferrell 1992; Porter 1994; Cowart 1995).

2. Be aware of whether determinations of concepts, such as appropriate pain behavior, patients' tolerance levels, and advantages and disadvantages of treatment alternatives, speak primarily to the needs of patients and their families or primarily to the needs of clinicians (Stein 1985; Geach 1987; Gadow 1989; Weissman and Haddox 1989; Roy 1992; Zussman 1992; Qiu 1993; Anderson and Anderson 1994; Somerville 1994; Walco et al. 1994; Shapiro 1995).

3. Be aware of the ways in which the social history of attitudes about pain and the medical history of assessment, treatment, and value of pain can affect current lay and professional attitudes about patients with pain (Scarry 1985; Vrancken 1989; Macrae et al. 1992; Max 1992; Cunningham 1993; Anderson and Anderson 1994; Porter 1994; Somerville 1994; Walco et al. 1994).

4. Understand the difference between informed consent in clinical treatment and in research, as well as the moral importance of both (Levine 1988; Brody 1992; Zussman 1992). Be aware of effective ways to involve patients and their families in the pain assessment and treatment process (Acute Pain Management Guideline Panel 1992c; American Cancer Society and National Cancer Institute 1992; Jacox et al. 1994b; McGrath et al. 1994; Miaskowski 1994).

B. Vulnerable groups

1. Understand the vulnerability of patients who cannot talk at all or who have limited ability to communicate verbally, including infants and children, the elderly, and those treated in the emergency room, intensive care unit, or nursing homes. Understand the professional responsibility to use, for assessment purposes, multiple forms of nonverbal indicators that may communicate pain (Acute Pain Management Guideline Panel 1992a; Melding 1992; Shapiro and Ferrell 1992; Cunningham 1993; Jacox et al. 1994a; Somerville 1994; Shapiro 1995).

2. Understand the vulnerability of patients with diseases such as cancer or conditions such as burns, where there has been a historical, professional acceptance of severe, unremitting pain (Bonica 1953; Max 1992; Cowart 1995). Know (1) the distinctions among psychological dependence (addiction), physical dependence, and tolerance; (2) the causes of pseudo-addiction;

and (3) common fears and confusions about opioid pain control (Weissman and Haddox 1989; Acute Pain Management Guideline Panel 1992b; Jacox et al. 1994a; Walco et al. 1994).

3. Understand the vulnerability of dying patients or others with serious conditions, who prefer death over life because their pain is not adequately controlled (Jacox et al. 1994a; Somerville 1994; Cowart 1995). Be aware that the acceptability of physician-assisted suicide may be related to lack of knowledge of effective means of pain control or lack of actual availability of these methods (Foley 1991, 1995). Understand the ethical principle of "double effect," as it applies to pain control. (It is acceptable to provide medication for pain control, which has as a secondary effect hastening death, when the primary intention is to provide adequate pain control that can be provided in no other manner.) (Council on Ethical and Judicial Affairs 1992; John Paul II 1995).

4. Understand the vulnerability of chronic pain patients, especially as it may be related to the mystery and complexity of the condition, and the clinician's wish for simple diagnoses and treatment (Vrancken 1989; Melding 1992; Roy 1992; Shapiro 1995).

5. Understand the vulnerability of economically disadvantaged patients, and patients who live in locations where laws (as part of the war on drugs) restrict the use of opioids, even to patients in need. Understand the principle of justice, as it applies to providing fair access to health care, especially pain control (Cunningham 1993; Foley 1994; Jacox et al. 1994a).

C. Quality assurance

1. Be aware of the institutional, as well as unit and individual, moral responsibility for providing appropriate pain care, and the consequent need for an interdisciplinary, system-wide approach that acknowledges the physiological and psychological complexity of pain (Mount 1990; Acute Pain Management Guideline Panel 1992a; Acute Pain Management Guideline Panel 1992b; Max 1992; Jacox et al. 1994a;. Miaskowski 1994).

2. Understand that current, local standards of care may be far from ideal and that efforts to change standards must involve changes in moral awareness and commitment, as well as changes in the technical education of professionals (Melzack 1988; Mount 1990; Macrae et al. 1992; Max 1992; Carr 1993; Cunningham 1993; Jacox et al. 1994a).

III. Research

A. Statements of research ethics

1. Know the standards provided in international, national, and professional statements of biomedical research ethics, including instances where standards conflict with one another (Levine 1988; World Medical Association 1989; CIOMS and WHO 1993; Mariner 1993; McNeill 1993; Gorlin 1994; International Association for the Study of Pain, in press).

2. Understand that laws or rules, traditions, and resources within particular societies and medical cultures may make these standards only partly applicable, or difficult to apply (CIOMS and WHO 1993; Qiu 1993; CIOMS 1995).

B. Research design, review, and implementation

1. Understand that ethical research requires sound methods, but sound methods do not guarantee ethical research; researchers are responsible for the well-being of subjects even when subjects or their proxies have given consent (Silverman 1985; World Medical Association 1989; CIOMS and WHO 1993; McGrath 1993; Rothman and Michels 1994; International Association for the Study of Pain, in press)

2. Understand philosophical arguments for and against randomized, controlled trials (Silverman 1985; Nicholson 1986; Gifford 1994), including the use of placebo controls, when effective forms of pain prevention or control are already scientifically proven (Rothman and Michels 1994), or when the subjects receiving placebos have absent or such diminished cognitive capacity (such as infants or comatose patients) that they have no possibility of positive placebo effect.

3. Be aware that, as a matter of justice, the requirement not to exceed the subject's tolerance limit applies equally to situations of experimentally induced pain and to situations of research about pain that is consequent to disease, injury, or medical procedures (Loewy 1991; International Association for the Study of Pain, in press).

4. Understand benefits, appropriate use, standard methodologies, and ethical concerns of qualitative research about pain (Agar 1986; Ramos 1989; Zussman 1992).

5. Be aware that the complex nature of pain and the common use of interdisciplinary teams for clinical practice do not contradict the ethical requirement that particular research projects be carried out only by scientifically qualified persons (World Medical Association 1989; CIOMS and WHO 1993).

6. Be aware of the necessity of independent ethical review committees and the possibility that even they may be adversely affected by factors such as reputation of proposed principal investigators, traditional medical acceptability of certain levels of pain in subjects, funding needs of the research institution, or the lack of adequate subject representation on the committee (Cunningham and Hutchinson 1990; McNeill 1993).

7. Be aware of potential problems of unfair profit or scientific bias due to the priorities of the research funding source, whether that source is institutional, commercial, private nonprofit, or government (CIOMS and WHO 1993; Korenman 1993; McNeill 1993).

C. Informed consent

1. Understand the key characteristics of informed consent; it must be legally competent, voluntary, informed, and with understanding (Levine 1988; CIOMS and WHO 1993). Be aware of acknowledged and unacknowledged difficulties of obtaining informed consent for research (Silverman 1985; Cunningham and Hutchinson 1990; Mariner 1993; McNeill 1993; Meslin 1993).

2. Be aware that, in some countries, dignity and autonomy of the subject, which researchers protect with informed consent, cannot be separated from that of the family or community (Cunningham and Hutchinson 1990; CIOMS and WHO 1993; Qiu 1993).

3. Be aware that those groups of persons who are vulnerable in the clinical context may also be vulnerable in the research context because they cannot give voluntary consent (Silverman 1985; Shapiro and Ferrell 1992). Additional groups might include prisoners, the mentally ill, students,

research center employees, or those who generally have limited access to health care (Levine 1988; CIOMS and WHO 1993; Korenman 1993).

4. Be aware that some groups, such as children or pregnant women, are vulnerable to unfair exclusion from pain research (CIOMS and WHO 1993).

5 Understand that some groups may be exploitable, in addition to or instead of vulnerable, because they can be misused. Subjects in externally sponsored research projects may be at special risk (CIOMS and WHO 1993; Mariner 1993; Qiu 1993).

6. Be aware of the elements of providing complete information to subjects or their proxies, including treatment options for pain prevention and control available for patients who are treated outside the research project or institution (CIOMS and WHO 1993; Rothman and Michels 1994; International Association for the Study of Pain, in press).

7. Understand that it is morally important to consider from the subjects' point of view the actual benefits, harms, and costs to subjects, as well as potential risks to them, in addition to considering the medical experts' evaluation of these factors (Nicholson 1986; Cunningham and Hutchinson 1990). Be aware of both the subjective and objective nature of the risk, harm, and benefit evaluation by both clinicians and researchers (Meslin 1993).

D. Animals

1. Be aware of the history and continuing influence of the scientific belief that animals do not experience pain, despite their physiological and behavioral signs of pain. Understand the similarity between this history and the history of medical treatment of groups of human patients who cannot talk (Rollin 1990; Cunningham 1993).

2. Know the standards for sound animal pain research, including attention to their physiological and mental health (International Association for the Study of Pain 1983; Dubner 1989).

3. Know the ethical standards for animal pain research (International Association for the Study of Pain 1983; Rollin 1990), understanding that no group of humans should receive less protection than animals receive (Stang et al. 1988).

REFERENCES

Acute Pain Management Guideline Panel, Acute Pain Management in Infants, Children, and Adolescents: Operative and Medical Procedures, Quick Reference Guide for Clinicians, AHCPR Pub. No. 92-0020, Agency for Health Care Policy and Research, Public Health Service, U.S. Department of Health and Human Services, Rockville, MD, 1992a.

Acute Pain Management Guideline Panel, Acute Pain Management: Operative or Medical Procedures and Trauma, Clinical Practice Guideline, AHCPR Pub. No. 92-0032, Agency for Health Care Policy and Research, Public Health Service, U.S. Department of Health and Human Services, Rockville, MD, 1992b.

Acute Pain Management Guideline Panel, Pain Control After Surgery: A Patient's Guide, AHCPR Pub. No. 92-0021, Agency for Health Care Policy and Research, Public Health Service, U.S. Department of Health and Human Services, Rockville, MD, 1992c.

Agar, M., Speaking of Ethnography, Sage Publications, Beverly Hills, CA, 1986.

American Cancer Society and National Cancer Institute, Questions and Answers About Pain Control: A Guide For People with Cancer and Their Families, American Cancer Society, Atlanta, 1992.

Anderson, R.T. and Anderson, S.T., Culture and pain. In: F.A. Djite-Bruce (Trans.), The Puzzle of Pain, Gordon and Breach Arts International, East Roseville, NSW, 1994, pp. 120–138.

Bonica, J.J. (Ed.), The Management of Pain, Lea & Febiger, Philadelphia, 1953.

Brody, H., The Healer's Power, Yale University Press, New Haven, 1992.

Carr, D.B., Pain control: the new "whys" and "hows," Pain Clinical Updates, 1 (1993) 1–4, newsletter, IASP, Seattle.

Cassell, E.J., Treating the patient's subjective state, Pain Forum, 4 (1995) 186–188.

Council for International Organizations of Medical Sciences (CIOMS) and World Health Organization (WHO), International Ethical Guidelines for Biomedical Research Involving Human Subjects, CIOMS, Geneva, 1993.

Council for International Organizations of Medical Sciences (CIOMS), A global agenda for bioethics: Declaration of Ixtapa, IASP Newsletter Jan/Feb (1995) 4–6.

Council on Ethical and Judicial Affairs, American Medical Association, Decisions near the end of life, JAMA, 267 (1992) 2229–2233.

Cowart, D.S., Confronting death in one's own way, Pain Forum, 4 (1995) 179–181.

Cunningham, N., Moral and ethical issues in clinical practice. In: K.J.S. Anand and P.J. McGrath (Eds.), Pain in Neonates, Elsevier Science Publishers B.V., Amsterdam, 1993, pp. 255–273.

Cunningham, N. and Hutchinson, S., Neonatal nurses and issues in research ethics, Neonatal Network, 8 (1990) 29–47.

Dubner, R., Methods of assessing pain in animals. In: P.D. Wall and R. Melzack (Eds.), Textbook of Pain, Churchill Livingstone, Edinburgh, 1989, pp. 247–256.

Foley, K.M., The relationship of pain and symptom management to patient requests for physician-assisted suicide, J. Pain Sympt. Manage., 6 (1991) 289–297.

Foley, K.M., The World Health Organization Program in Cancer Pain Relief and Palliative Care. In: G.F. Gebhart, D.L. Hammond, and T.S. Jensen (Eds.), Proceedings of the 7th World Congress on Pain, Progress in Pain Research and Management, Vol. 2, IASP Press, Seattle, 1994, pp. 59–74.

Foley, K.M., Pain, physician-assisted suicide and euthanasia, Pain Forum, 4 (1995) 163–178.

Gadow, S., Remembered in the body: pain and moral uncertainty. In: L.D. Kliever (Ed.), Dax's Case: Essays in Medical Ethics and Human Meaning, Southern Methodist University Press, Dallas, 1989, pp. 151–167.

Geach, B., Pain and coping. Image: Journal of Nursing Scholarship, 19 (1987) 12–15.

Gifford, F., The conflict between randomized clinical trials and the therapeutic obligation. In: E. Erwin, S. Gendin, and L. Kleiman (Eds.), Ethical Issues in Scientific Research: An Anthology, Garland Publishing, Inc., New York, 1994, pp. 179–200.

Gorlin, R.A., (Ed.), Codes of Professional Responsibility, 3rd ed., Bureau of National Affairs, Inc., Washington, DC, 1994.

Hilberg, R. Perpetrators, Victims, Bystanders: The Jewish Catastrophe 1933–1945, Aaron Asher Books, New York, 1992.

Institute of Medicine, Child Health and Human Rights: An Address by James P. Grant, National Academy Press, Washington, DC, 1994.

International Association for the Study of Pain, Ethical guidelines for investigations of experimental pain in conscious animals, Pain, 16 (1983) 109–110.

International Association for the Study of Pain, Ethical guidelines for pain research in humans, Pain, in press.

Jacox, A., Carr, D.B., Payne, R., et al., Management of Cancer Pain, Clinical Practice Guideline No. 9, AHCPR Publication No. 94-0592, Agency for Health Care Policy and Research, U.S. Department of Health and Human Services, Public Health Service, Rockville, MD, 1994a.

Jacox, A., Carr, D.B., Payne, R., et al., Managing Cancer Pain, Patient Guide, Consumer Version, Clinical Practice Guideline No. 9, AHCPR Publication No. 94-0595, Agency for Health Care Policy and Research, U.S. Department of Health and Human Services, Public Health Service, Rockville, MD, 1994b.

John Paul II, Pope, The Gospel of Life: Evangelium Vitae, Times Books, New York, 1995.

Korenman, S.G., Conflicts of interest and commercialization of research, Acad. Med., 68 (1993) S18–S22.

Krystal, H., Trauma: considerations of its intensity and chronicity. In: H. Krystal and W.G. Niederland (Eds.), Psychic Traumatization: Aftereffects in Individuals and Communities, Little, Brown & Co., Boston, 1971, pp. 11–28.

Levine, R.J., Ethics and Regulation of Clinical Research, 2nd ed., Yale University Press, New Haven, 1988.

Loewy, E.H., Suffering and the Beneficent Community: Beyond Libertarianism, State University of New York Press, Albany, 1991.

Macrae, W.A., Davies, H.T.O. and Crombie, I.K. Pain: paradigms and treatments, Pain, 49 (1992) 289–291.

Mariner, W.K., Distinguishing "exploitable" from "vulnerable" populations: when consent is not the issue. In: Z. Bankowski and R.J. Levine (Eds.), Ethics and Research on Human Subjects: International Guidelines, Proceedings of the XXVIth CIOMS Conference, Geneva, Switzerland, 5-7 February 1992, Council for International Organizations of Medical Sciences, Geneva, 1993, pp. 44–55.

Max, M.B., Improving outcomes of analgesic treatment: is education enough? IASP Newsletter, Nov/Dec (1992), 2–6.

McGrath, P.A. Inducing pain in children: a controversial issue, Pain, 52 (1993) 255–257.

McGrath, P.J., Finley, G.A. and Ritchie, J., Pain, Pain, Go Away: Helping Children With Pain, Association for the Care of Children's Health, Bethesda, MD, 1994.

McNeill, P.M., The Ethics and Politics of Human Experimentation, Cambridge University Press, Cambridge, 1993.

Melding, P.S., Psychosocial aspects of chronic pain and the elderly, IASP Newsletter, Jan/Feb (1992) 2–4.

Melzack, R., The tragedy of needless pain: a call for social action. In: R. Dubner, G.F. Gebhart and M.R. Bond (Eds.), Proceedings of the Vth World Congress on Pain, Pain Research and Clinical Management, Vol. 3, Elsevier, Amsterdam, 1988, pp. 1–11.

Meslin, E.M., Philosophical considerations about risk and risk assessment in medical research. In: G. Koren (Ed.), Textbook of Ethics in Pediatric Research, Krieger Publishing Company, Malabar, FL, 1993, pp. 37–55.

Miaskowski, C., Effective cancer pain management: from guidelines to quality improvement, Pain Clinical Updates, 2 (1994) 1–4, newsletter, IASP, Seattle.

Mount, E., Professional Ethics in Context: Institutions, Images and Empathy, Westminster/John Knox Press, Louisville, KY, 1990.

Nicholson, R.H. (Ed.), Medical Research with Children: Ethics, Law and Practice, Oxford University Press, Oxford, 1986.

Porter, R., Pain and history in the western world. In: F.A. Djite-Bruce (Trans.), The Puzzle of Pain, Gordon and Breach Arts International, East Roseville, NSW, 1994, pp. 98–119.

Qiu, R., Asian perspectives: tension between modern values and Chinese culture. In: Z. Bankowski and R.J. Levine (Eds.), Ethics and Research on Human Subjects: International Guidelines, Proceedings of the XXVIth CIOMS Conference, Geneva, Switzerland, 5-7 February 1992, Council for International Organizations of Medical Sciences, Geneva, 1993, pp. 188–197.

Ramos, M.C., Some ethical implications of qualitative research, Res. Nur. Health, 12 (1989) 57–63.

Randall, G.R. and Lutz, E.L., Serving Survivors of Torture: A Practical Manual for Health Professionals and Other Service Providers, American Association for the Advancement of Science, Washington, DC, 1991.

Rollin, B.E., The Unheeded Cry: Animal Consciousness, Animal Pain and Science, Oxford University Press, Oxford, 1990.

Rothman, K.J. and Michels, K.B., The continuing unethical use of placebo controls. N. Engl. J. Med., 331 (1994) 394–398.

Roy, R., The Social Context of the Chronic Pain Sufferer, University of Toronto Press, Toronto, 1992.

Scarry, E., The Body in Pain: The Making and Unmaking of the World, Oxford University Press, New York, 1985.

Schrag, C.O., Being in pain. In: V. Kestenbaum (Ed.), The Humanity of the Ill: Phenomenological Perspectives, The University of Tennessee Press, Knoxville, 1982, pp. 101–124.

Shapiro, B.S., The suffering of children and their families. In: B.R. Ferrell (Ed.), Suffering: Human Dimensions of Pain and Illness, Jones & Bartlett Publishers, Boston, 1995.

Shapiro, B.S. and Ferrell, B.R., Pain in children and the frail elderly: similarities and implications, APS Bulletin, Oct/Nov (1992) 11–13.

Silverman, W.A., Human Experimentation: A Guided Step into the Unknown, Oxford University Press, Oxford, 1985.

Somerville, M.A., Death of pain: pain, suffering, and ethics. In: G.F. Gebhart, D.L. Hammond, and T.S. Jensen (Eds.), Proceedings of the 7th World Congress on Pain, Progress in Pain Research and Management, Vol. 2, IASP Press, Seattle, 1994, pp. 41–58.

Stang, H.J., Gunnar, M.R., Snellman, L., Condon, L.M. and Kestenbaum, R., Local anesthesia for neonatal circumcision: effects on distress and cortisol response, JAMA, 259 (1988) 1507–1511.

Stein, H.F., On healing and suffering. In: H.F. Stein and M. Apprey (Eds.), Context and Dynamics in Clinical Knowledge, University Press of Virginia, Charlottesville, 1985, pp. 198–210.

U.N. Commission on Human Rights, Universal Declaration of Human Rights, United Nations, New York, 1948.

Vrancken, M.A.E., Schools of thought on pain, Pain, 29 (1989) 435–444.

Walco, G.A., Cassidy, R.C., and Schechter, N.L., Pain, hurt, and harm: the ethics of pain control in infants and children. N. Engl. J. Med., 331 (1994) 541–544.

Weissman, D.E. and Haddox, J.D., Opioid pseudoaddiction: an iatrogenic syndrome, Pain, 36 (1989) 363–366.

World Medical Association, World Medical Association Declaration of Helsinki: Recommendations Guiding Physicians in Biomedical Research Involving Human Subjects, 1964, revised in Hong Kong, 1989.

Zussman, R., Intensive Care: Medical Ethics and the Medical Profession, University of Chicago Press, Chicago, 1992.